BRAIN CT

An Introduction

John R. Bradshaw

BA, MB, BCh, DMRD, FRCR, FRCP(C)
*Consultant Neuroradiologist Frenchay Hospital,
Bristol*

WRIGHT
Bristol 1985

Published by:
John Wright & Sons Ltd, Techno House, Redcliffe Way, Bristol BS1 6NX, England.

British Library Cataloguing in Publication Data

Bradshaw, John R.
  Brain CT : an introduction.
  1. Brain—Radiography   2. Tomography
  I. Title
  612'.82   RC386.6.T64

ISBN 0 7236 0855 5

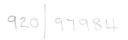

Computer Typeset by
Kestrel Data, Exeter, Devon EX2 7JQ.

Printed in Great Britain by
John Wright & Sons (Printing) Ltd at the Stonebridge Press, Bristol BS4 5NU.

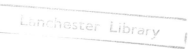

Preface

The development of computed tomography (CT) by Godfrey Hounsfield and EMI in 1972 earned him the Nobel Prize and changed for all time the investigation of brain pathology. Prior to that time detailed radiological assessment of the brain required uncomfortable and potentially dangerous techniques such as air-encephalography and cerebral angiography. The former is now practically obsolete and the latter required far less often. Furthermore, the CT scan provides us with anatomical and pathological detail not possible by other techniques short of craniotomy, and in most cases further major diagnostic procedures are not required. The benefits for patients and those whose duty it is to care for them are beyond measure. It is now generally recognized to be one of the greatest advances in diagnosis since the discovery of X-rays.

There are now thousands of CT scanners scattered throughout many countries of the world, and most doctors come into contact with such an instrument or its images at some time in their career. This book aims to provide an introduction to the CT brain scan, and the pathology it may reveal. The cases used have been gathered over a two-year period in a busy regional neurosciences unit. The style of presentation has been carefully chosen to appeal to a wide variety of readers including: student and qualified radiologists, other clinicians of both consultant and junior status, nurses, radiographers, etc. Detailed discussions of physics and techniques have been omitted, as these aspects have been well covered elsewhere.

I am indebted to my colleagues at Frenchay Hospital for their forbearance during this project and in particular to Dr Gordon Thomson for much encouragement and advice. I am also pleased to acknowledge cases from the CT scanning services at the Bristol Royal Infirmary, Cheltenham General Hospital and Gloucester Royal Hospital. My thanks are also due to the many radiographers who performed the scans to such high standards, and to Miss Sally Alden for her tireless work at the word processor.

Finally, this book is dedicated to my long-suffering family for their patience and support during a lengthy literary gestation.

Bristol, 1985   JRB

v

Contents

Introduction

Format

The book is divided into two parts. The first provides a simple introduction to how the scan is produced and the appearance of a normal brain on the images obtained. A selection of artefacts and normal variants is included. In the second part a series of over eighty cases is presented, portraying the common pathology encountered in everyday clinical practice with a basic guide as to how this pathology is revealed on the scan. The cases are grouped together according to their appearance on the scan, e.g. the first thirteen cases show a range of conditions that are high density lesions, and do not enhance after contrast enhancement. (This group is followed by others including low density lesions, posterior fossa lesions, hydrocephalus, etc. The group to which the case belongs is identified at the top of each right-hand page.) This enables the reader to compare an actual clinical case with a spectrum of the common differential diagnoses for that appearance.

For readers wishing to study a particular broad topic, e.g. trauma, this presents many appearances, and is therefore represented in different sections for each of these appearances. The pathology index at the end of the book shows where such a topic is discussed in different cases.

Each case can also be used as a self-examining exercise by covering up the right-hand side of each page spread and attempting to make a diagnosis from the clinical data and the accompanying images on the left-hand page (images marked '+C' have been taken after contrast enhancement). The right-hand page gives the broad group of appearances to which the case belongs, and then the diagnosis followed by an analysis of the images and the differential diagnoses.

The analysis of lesions of the orbit, complex congenital brain abnormalities and high resolution multiplanar images of the pituitary fossa, etc. are beyond the scope of this book. A brief list of suggested further reading is given on page 196.

Throughout the manual a basic understanding of simple anatomical and pathological terms is assumed.

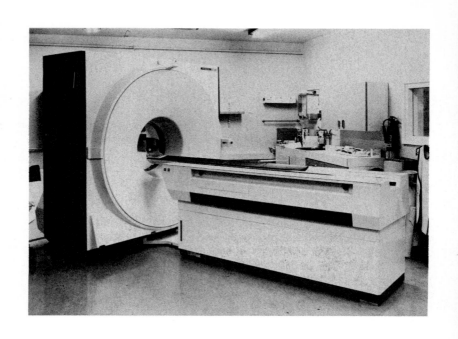

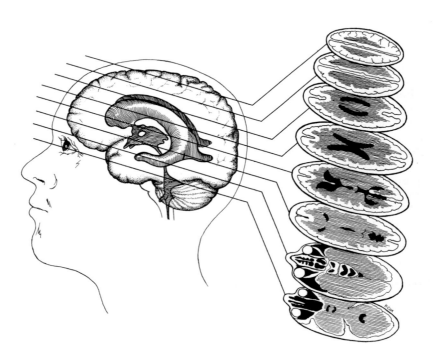

Image generation and display

CT brain scan images are produced by computerized re-
construction of a slice of head tissues which has been analysed by a
moving X-ray beam. The patient lies comfortably on a couch with his
head in the aperture of the gantry. This contains the X-ray tube and
detectors which generate digital information from each slice. This
digital information is then processed by the computer to produce the
images. Depending on·the machine each slice takes from 10 to 60 se-
conds to examine, and a full routine examination about 20 to 60
minutes. The procedure is quite painless, but some patients may
require a further set of 'enhanced' scans after an intravenous
injection of an iodinated contrast medium (similar to that used in
intravenous urography). Introduction of air or contrast medium into
the subarachnoid spaces or ventricles may also be used to provide
further information in certain special situations. These techniques are
beyond the scope of this book. Most modern scanners can also per-
form body scans.

Each image represents a slice of brain tissue and these are presented in sequence from the base of the brain upwards. A slice is usually 5-10 mm thick and normally touches its companion cuts on either
side so that reviewing a sequence of slices in order enables one to
build up a mental picture of the whole brain. The standard position of
the slices and their visual sequence are shown. Many modern
machines are capable of scanning (or recalculating the data) into
other planes, e.g. sagittal or coronal.

The image and its densities

The CT brain scan is capable of displaying all the range of densities between air and bone, indeed this range is present on most images in clinical use. Air is shown as black and bone as white, with all the intervening densities as varying shades of grey. The values of grey can be adjusted by varying the settings on the imaging system known as window width and level. But for most purposes and throughout this book the settings used are constant to avoid confusion.

The densities encountered on the majority of scans include the following (their approximate numerical values in Hounsfield units are given):

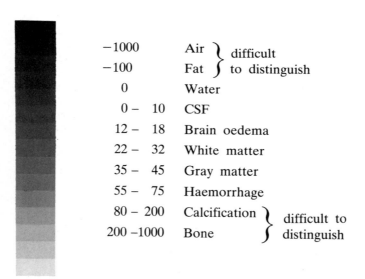

−1000	Air	} difficult
−100	Fat	to distinguish
0	Water	
0 − 10	CSF	
12 − 18	Brain oedema	
22 − 32	White matter	
35 − 45	Gray matter	
55 − 75	Haemorrhage	
80 − 200	Calcification	} difficult to
200 −1000	Bone	distinguish

The CT images reproduced here are mostly from two machines, the EMI 1010 Head Scanner and an up-to-date GE 8800 Body Scanner. Most of the conditions shown can be readily diagnosed on quite basic CT scanners. All scans are displayed with the patient's left side on the left of the image and the face at the top. Images showing '+C' represent a contrast-enhanced scan.

Scan supervision and interpretation

Special preparations are not required for most patients having brain scans. Patients should however be kept fasting for 4 hours prior to the scan as some will require an injection of iodinated contrast medium (contrast enhancement) and this may produce some nausea. All patients should be reassured and the procedure explained to them; restless or unco-operative patients will probably require sedation.

The indications for CT brain scanning are numerous and include: suspected head injury, tumour, stroke, infarct, intracranial infection, hydrocephalus, etc. Scanning of epileptic patients and those with dementia will reveal underlying pathology in many cases. The extent to which such problems can be evaluated by CT is governed by available resources.

The standard unenhanced scan should produce 8–10 consecutive slices of 8–10 mm thickness from the lower posterior fossa to the vertex and these images should be assessed for any lesion, and to see if any area of brain has been omitted. Most focal lesions need to be enhanced as do most patients with suspected metastases, orbit, pituitary or posterior fossa lesions. The purpose of enhancement is to improve the pick-up rate of lesions and to provide further information about lesions that are visible on the plain scan. Contrast enhancement usually involves a bolus intravenous injection of a suitable iodinated contrast medium. In some departments this is given by infusion. After this the scan series is repeated. The contrast medium renders many vascular structures visible and causes many lesions to show increased density in specific patterns. This is due to the presence of multiple small abnormal vessels in many lesions and/or a breakdown in the blood-brain barrier allowing the dense contrast material to enter the lesion. The plain scan effects of lesions include dilatation of one or more ventricles (hydrocephalus), compression or displacement of those ventricles and midline structures (mass effect). The lesions themselves may be the same density as brain (isodense), or of higher or lower density than brain. The position of a lesion, its density, its effects on surrounding structures and its pattern of enhancement together with clinical details all help to provide facts on which a probable diagnosis can be based. These aspects are covered throughout the case discussions.

It must be clearly understood that contrast enhancement, like intravenous urography, carries a small but significant risk and should only be given where clear indications for its use exist.

It must be emphasized that brain disorders, like most other things in nature, do not always conform to the rules and the diagnosis may not be 'cast-iron' from the scans. Follow-up scans are very helpful in clarifying the situation, as the progress of a lesion over a period of time is usually an index of its character.

Anatomy

The anatomical features shown on any particular slice depend on a number of factors including: the thickness and position of the slice, the angulation of the head during that slice and the quality of the scanner. The following illustrations show fairly typical slices of 10 mm thickness, consecutively arranged from the skull base to the vertex. The head angulation used was standard at about 15 degrees to the cantho-meatal line. The images were generated on a state of the art scanner (GE 8800) and represent quality close to the maximum possible with current technology. Only the important anatomical structures are identified, as detailed anatomical analysis is beyond the scope of this book. Variation of the head angulation will include different combinations of structures on individual slices, other than those shown here. Thinner slices help to reduce artefacts and give finer detail. These are particularly useful in the posterior fossa, sella turcica and orbit. Coronal and sagittal images, either directly produced or from reformatting of axial scan data, are beyond the scope of this book. A short section on some common normal variants and artefacts follows the anatomical images. Anatomy images XI and XII show some anatomical features visible on contrast enhanced scans.

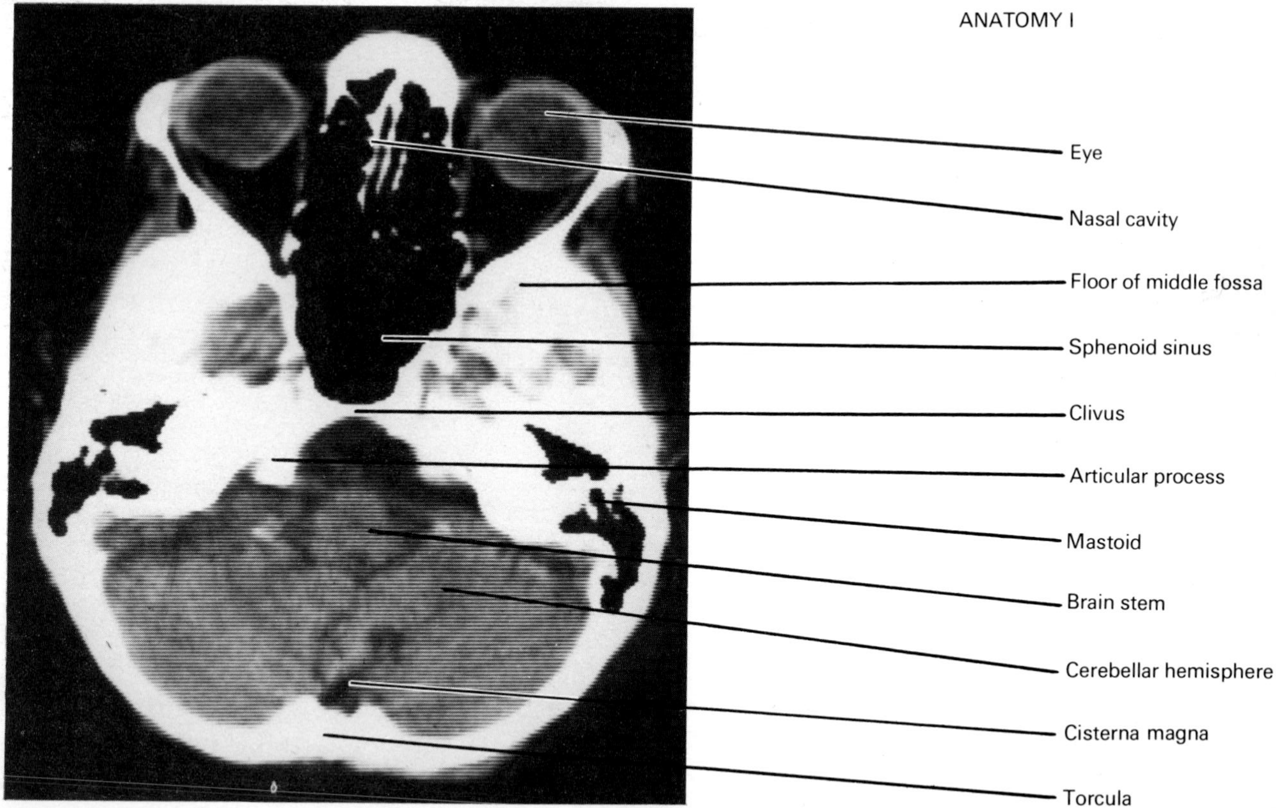

Eye

Nasal cavity

Floor of middle fossa

Sphenoid sinus

Clivus

Articular process

Mastoid

Brain stem

Cerebellar hemisphere

Cisterna magna

Torcula

ANATOMY II

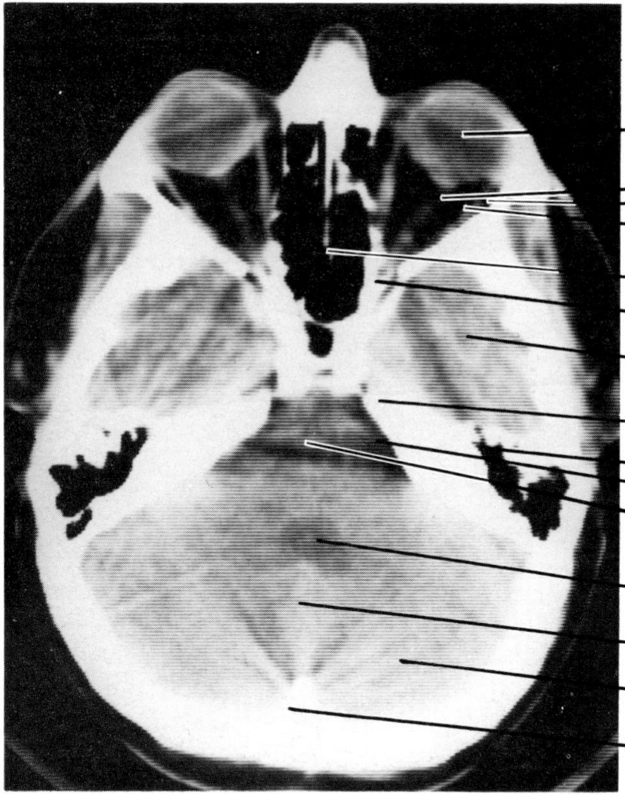

Eye
Optic nerve
Lateral rectus muscle
Retro-orbital fat
Nasal cavity/ethmoids
Optic foramen
Anterior temporal lobe
Petrous bone
Mastoid air cells
Cerebello-pontine angle
Brain stem
Fourth ventricle
Vermis
Cerebellar hemisphere
Torcula

ANATOMY III

Nasal cavity
Upper orbit
Olfactory/frontal lobes
Ethmoids
Greater wing of sphenoid
Orbital fissure
Tuberculum sellae
Anterior clinoid
Pituitary fossa
Temporal lobe
Dorsum sellae
Brain stem
Upper petrous bone (ridge)
Upper fourth ventricle
Vermis
Cerebellar hemisphere

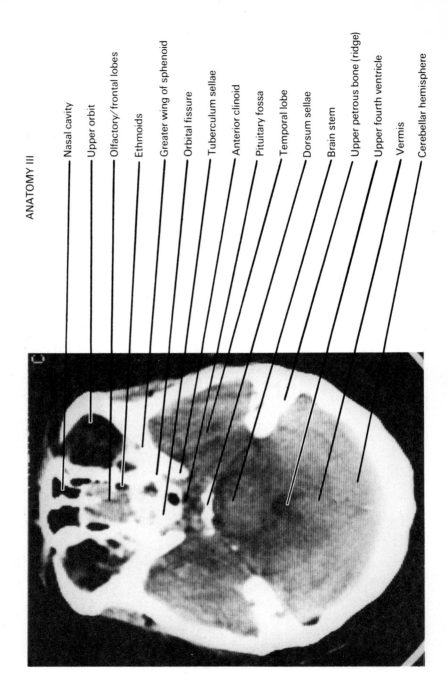

ANATOMY IV

Anterior interhemispheral fissure
Frontal lobe
Lateral sphenoid ridge
Sylvian fissure
Suprasellar cistern
Temporal lobe
Temporal horn
Ambient cistern
Brain stem
Lateral petrous ridge
Upper fourth ventricle
Vermis
Cerebellar hemisphere

ANATOMY V

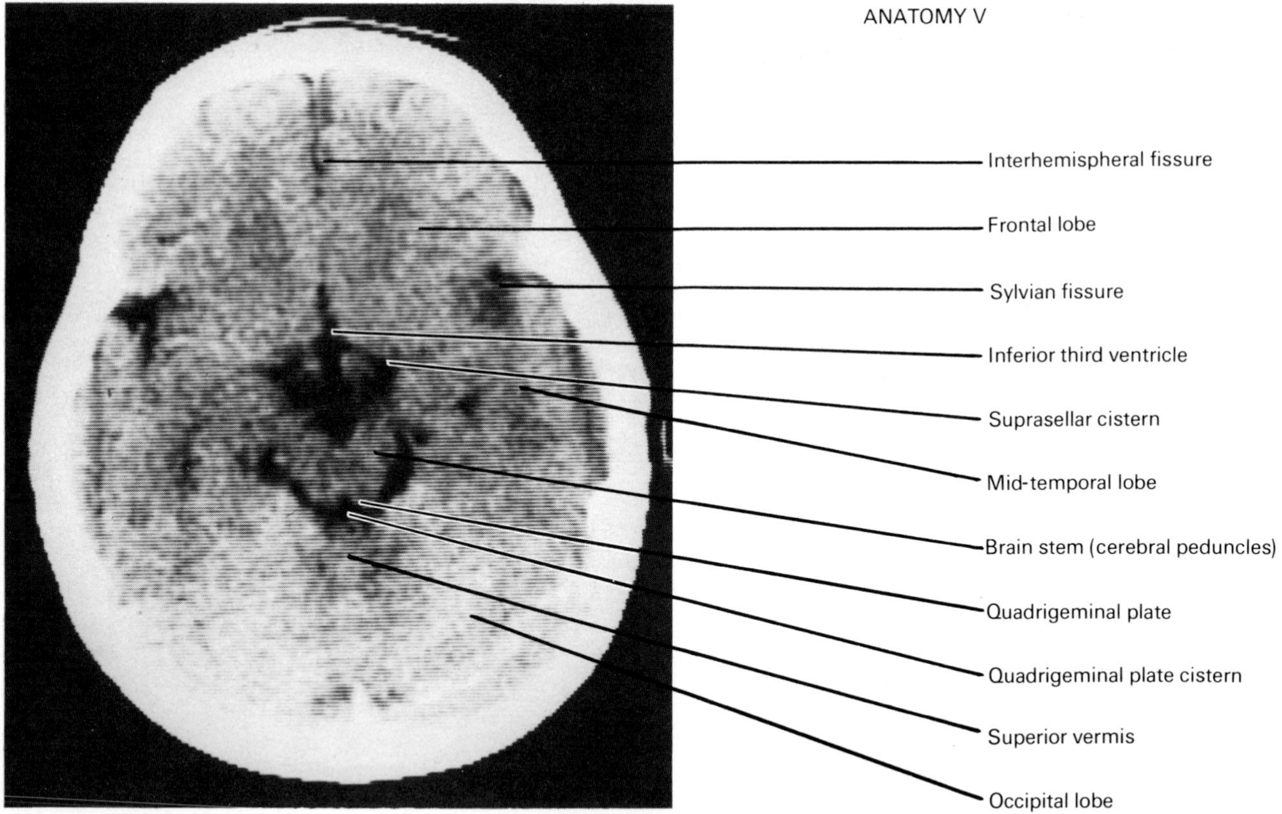

Interhemispheral fissure
Frontal lobe
Sylvian fissure
Inferior third ventricle
Suprasellar cistern
Mid-temporal lobe
Brain stem (cerebral peduncles)
Quadrigeminal plate
Quadrigeminal plate cistern
Superior vermis
Occipital lobe

12

ANATOMY VI

Interhemispheral fissure/falx
White matter frontal lobe
Genu (corpus callosum)
Frontal horn
Caudate nucleus
Anterior limb internal capsule
Lentiform nucleus
Sylvian fissure
Posterior limb internal capsule
Third ventricle
Thalamus
Pineal gland
Choroid plexus
Trigone (lateral ventricle)
Apex of vermis
Occipital lobe
Posterior falx

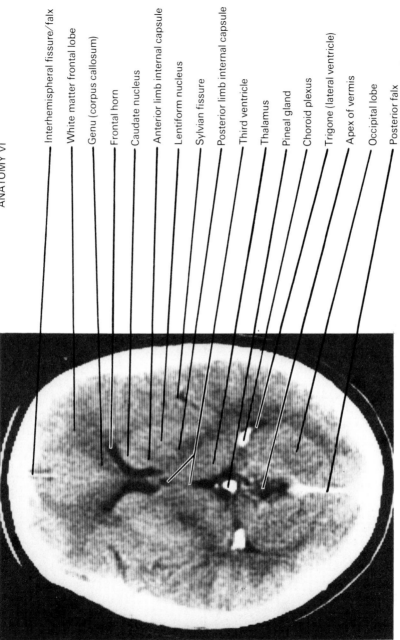

13

ANATOMY VII

Frontal lobe

Genu of corpus callosum

Lateral ventricle (body)

White matter

Choroid plexus

Parietal lobe

Splenium of corpus callosum

Grey matter (occipital lobe)

White matter (occipital lobe)

Posterior falx

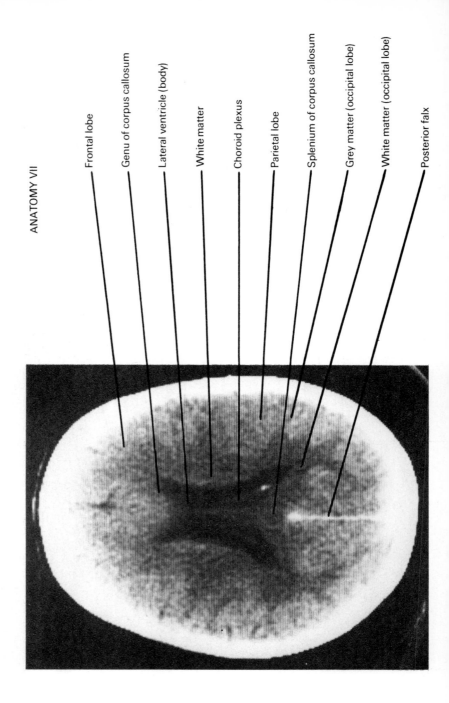

14

Anterior falx

Cortical sulci

Grey matter

Body of corpus callosum

Lateral ventricle

White matter

Posterior falx

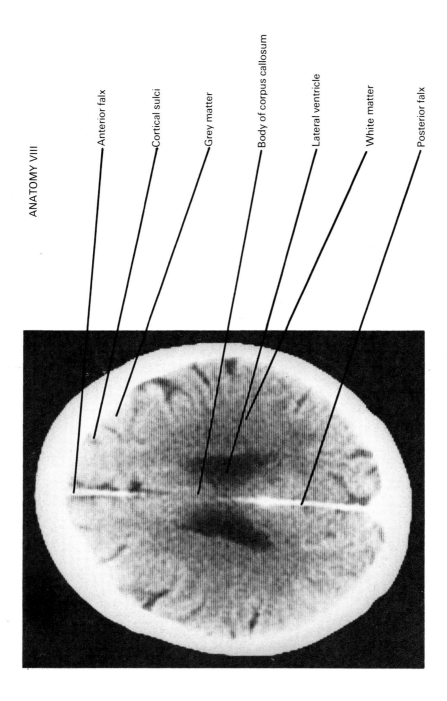

15

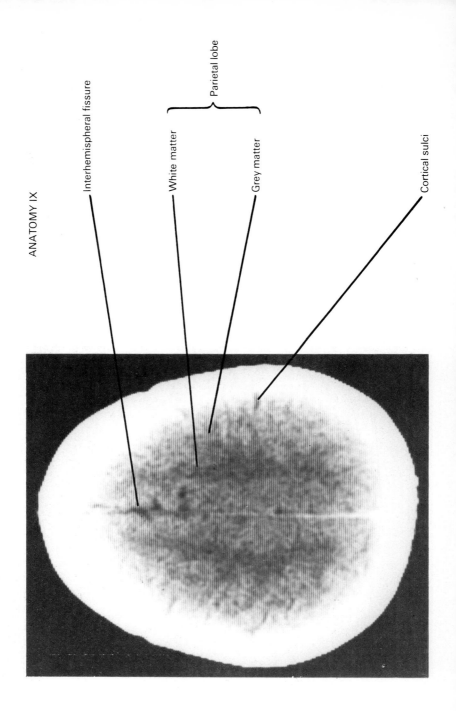

Interhemispheral fissure

Parietal lobe

White matter

Grey matter

Cortical sulci

Falx and interhemispheral fissure

Cortical sulci

ANATOMY XI

Anterior cerebral artery

Middle cerebral artery

Posterior communicating artery

Basilar artery

Posterior cerebral artery

Brain stem

Upper fourth ventricle

Cisterna magna

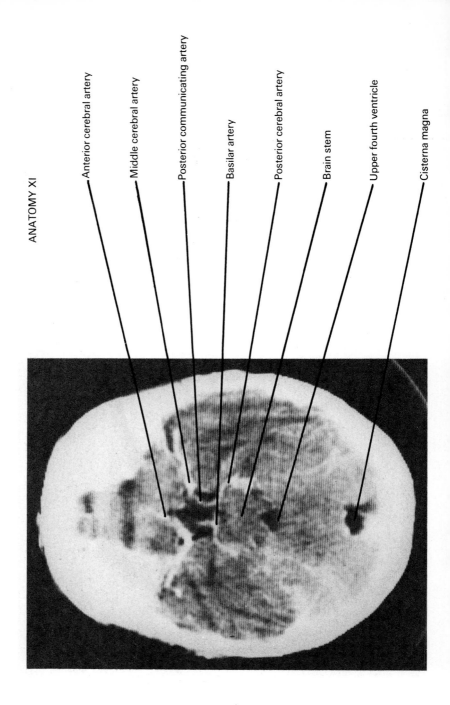

Anterior cerebral vessels

Enhancing choroid plexus

Middle cerebral vessels in sylvian fissure

Straight sinus

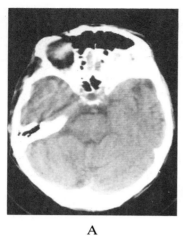

A

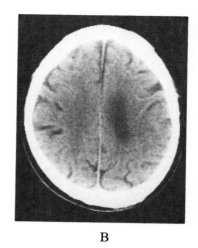

B

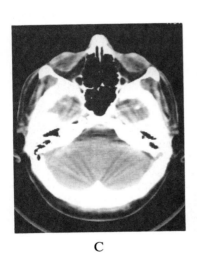

C

D

Artefacts and variants

XIII A. This scan shows asymmetry of the petrous bones. The one on the right is not visible. This is due to the patient not being properly placed in the scanner, with his head being tilted to one side. This is confirmed by the asymmetry of the orbits. The main importance of this artefact is that it makes cerebral structures look odd at higher levels.

B. The same patient as scan A with a scan through the upper ventricles showing how the asymmetrical placing of the head makes the brain look as though there is a mass effect in the left hemisphere. This pitfall can be avoided by routinely examining lower slices for evidence of asymmetry of the bony outlines.

C. Because of the high proportion of bone to brain in these low slices many images of the posterior fossa and middle fossae are impaired by streak artefacts. The horizontal black band between the petrous bones is common and is called a Hounsfield band. The radiating streaks from the torcula are also commonly seen. Both middle fossae also show diagonal band artefacts from the petrous bones.

D. The diagonal streaks across the whole head are due to a restless patient moving his head while the scan is being taken. This problem can usually be overcome by reassurance or adequate head fixation. Sedation may be required. This patient also has a congenitally large cisterna magna. This is of no consequence and not to be confused with a Dandy-Walker syndrome (*see* Case 74).

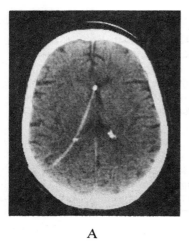

A

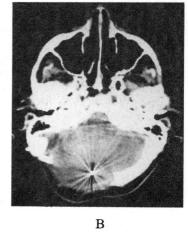

B

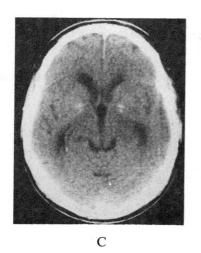

C

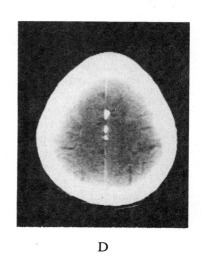

D

Artefacts and variants

XIV A. This scan shows a dense line running into the left lateral ventricle with a larger dense end in the frontal horn. This is a shunt tube inserted for the relief of hydrocephalus (successful!). It emerges through a burr hole in the parietal bone (not visible at this level). The appearance of these tubes is variable, but the position and density of this one are fairly typical.

B. A large bone defect is noted in the left side of the posterior fossa. This is due to previous surgery (craniotomy). A very dense artefact close to this and associated with radiating streaks is due to a piece of metal. Such densities may be the result of surgical clips or foreign bodies such as bullets. The contrast medium Myodil (Ethiodan) used in myelography often leaves small densities scattered in the basal cisterns.

C. There is symmetrical calcification in the basal nuclei. This is a normal finding in many people and is associated with increasing age. More florid examples, especially if associated with calcification in nuclei in the cerebellum, suggest a disorder of calcium metabolism (hypoparathyroidism).

D. Dense flecks or sheets of calcium are often seen in the falx. Less commonly, dura over the surface of the hemispheres may show sheets of calcification.

Case Studies

Case 1

Male, aged 69 years.

Severe frontal headache for 2 days. Known hypertensive.

Drowsy, confused.

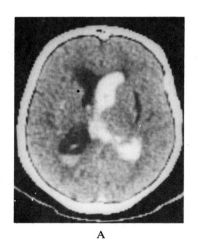

A

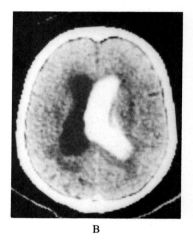

B

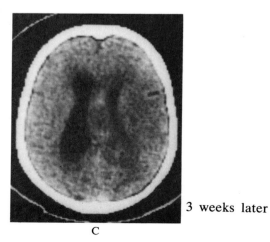

C

3 weeks later

Case 1

Spontaneous hypertensive haemorrhage

Scans A and B show raised density material in the right lateral ventricle and layering in the left occipital horn (scan A). Scan A also suggests that this haemorrhage may have originated from the right posterior thalamic region where there appears to be some blood outside the ventricle. There was no change after contrast enhancement. Scan C shows clearing of the haemorrhage 3 weeks later. Both ventricles are mildly dilated.

Fresh haemorrhage is the only pathology that looks quite like this. Calcification can be as white as this but the story of a sudden onset is quite typical. The high density of the haemorrhage reduces over a period of days or weeks and eventually leaves a low density area. Spontaneous haemorrhage is not uncommon in hypertensive patients and the thalamus and basal nuclei are common sites. Haemorrhages may also be the result of trauma, rupture of an aneurysm or an arterio-venous malformation (AVM), or bleeding from a tumour. Aneurysm haemorrhage usually has a subarachnoid component and lies along the line of major arteries (*see* Cases 4 and 5). Arteriovenous malformations (AVM) show serpiginous enhancement (*see* Case 15).

Illustrated below (scan D) the same pathology in the brain stem of a patient with a rapid deterioration in consciousness after a sudden onset of headache and brain stem signs.

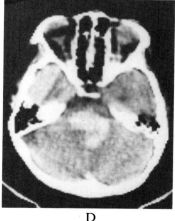

D

Case 2

Male, aged 25 years.

Drowsy following RTA. Blow on head. Headache.

Unco-operative. Consciousness impaired.

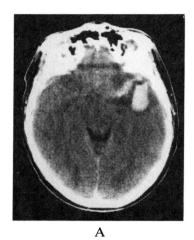

A

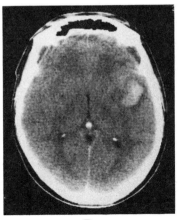

B

Case 2

Traumatic intra-cortical heomorrhage

Scans A and B show a high density lesion in the right temporal lobe; measurements showed this to be fresh blood. This is an unusual site for a hypertensive haemorrhage, but could be due to a ruptured aneurysm or AVM, although these usually show blood in the CSF (*see* Cases 3–5). Calcification can look like this but has higher density values. The story of a recent head injury confirms that this is traumatic in origin.

The scan below (scan C) shows a similar traumatic haemorrhage in the tip of the right frontal lobe. The frontal and temporal lobes are common sites for this intracortical type of haemorrhage due to impaction of the cortex into the box-like bony structures in these areas. Traumatic intracortical haemorrhage may, however, be found in any part of the brain including the brain stem.

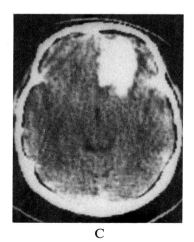

C

Case 3

Female, aged 20 years.

Sudden onset of severe headaches, drowsiness.

Semi comatose.

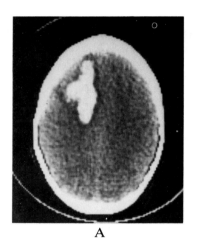

A

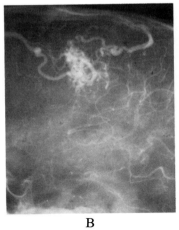

B

Case 3

Haemorrhage into AVM

Scan A shows a high density area in the upper left frontal lobe. Its appearance is similar to Cases 1 and 2. There was no change after enhancement. Because of the young age of the patient and the absence of a history of trauma or hypertension an underlying lesion should be excluded. Some small tumours and AVMs may not be visible on enhanced scans if haemorrhage has obscured the area, (*see* Case 16). Image B shows an arteriogram on this patient confirming the presence of an AVM within the area of haemorrhage.

AVMs are further discussed in Cases 15 and 56.

Case 4

Female, aged 45 years.

Sudden onset severe headache.

Drowsy, irritable.

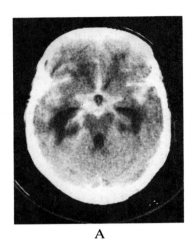

A

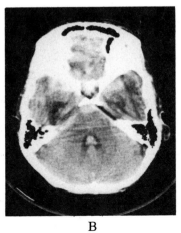

B

Case 4

Subarachnoid haemorrhage

Scan A shows a raised density area occupying the normally low density (CSF) area of the basal cisterns. The temporal horns are dilated indicating hydrocephalus. A similar density is also seen in the sylvian fissures. This is the typical appearance of blood mixed with the CSF in the basal cisterns. Because of the dilution by CSF it is usually less dense than intracerebral clot and may be quite difficult to see. It is visible for about 3–6 days after the bleed, so patients need to be scanned early if the diagnosis is suspected. The position of the blood may be helpful in locating the source of bleeding. Scan B shows blood in the fourth ventricle. Hydrocephalus is a common accompaniment of subarachnoid haemorrhage. Most of these subarachnoid haemorrhages are due to rupture of a berry aneurysm on the circle of Willis. The common sites are shown in diagram C together with the incidence of aneurysms at each site. Aneurysms may rupture wholly or partly into the cerebral substance.

An example of much more dilute blood staining of the CSF is shown in scan D where some blood is present in both sylvian fissures and the anterior interhemispheral fissure.

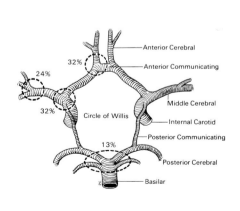

C

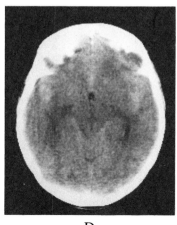

D

Case 5

Female, aged 34 years.

Sudden onset severe headache and neck stiffness.

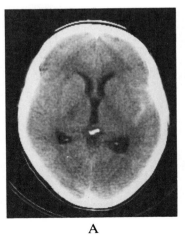

A

Case 5

Subarachnoid haemorrhage

Scan A shows irregular raised density in the right sylvian fissure. There was no change after contrast enhancement. This is due to blood in the sylvian fissure. Subarachnoid haemorrhage may be localized to the site of the bleed rather than spread throughout the CSF as in Case 4. This localization is usually a very good indication of the site of an aneurysm. In this case one would expect this to be on the right middle cerebral artery. A right carotid arteriogram (B) confirms this. Anterior localization of blood from an anterior communicating artery is shown in scan C.

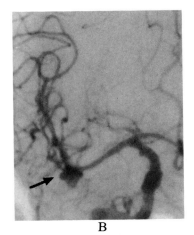

B

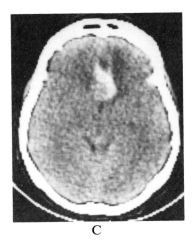

C

Case 6

Male, aged 20 years.

Deteriorating consciousness since head injury 24 hours ago.

Scalp wound and fracture right temporal area. Right hemiparesis.

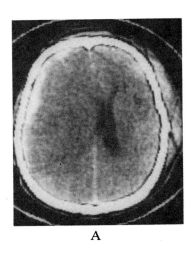

A

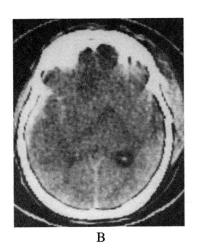

B

Case 6

Acute subdural haematoma

Scans A and B show swelling of the scalp over the right temporal region with an underlying fracture. The midline structures are displaced towards this side however and this fact together with the right hemiparesis leads one to suspect a lesion on the left. A shallow collection of blood is seen beneath the vault on the left covering much of the left hemisphere. Acute subdural haematomas are produced by tearing of veins crossing the subdural space and the site of the bleed may be some distance from the point of injury. The blood can spread freely in this space and presents as a shallow collection over most of the hemisphere. As the blood is resorbed its density gets less and the haematoma becomes indistinguishable from brain (*see* Case 36) and eventually of lower density than brain (Case 28).

Such lesions lie 'outside' the brain but may be associated with intracortical haemorrhage.

Case 7

Female, aged 36 years.

RTA. Briefly concussed—recovered.

Now deteriorating rapidly.

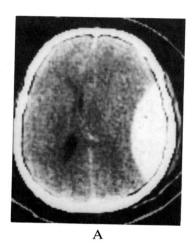

A

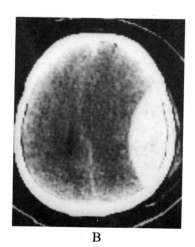

B

Case 7

Acute extra-dural haematoma

Scans A and B show a lens-shaped collection of blood in the right parietal area. There is midline shift to the left and compression of the right lateral ventricle. This appearance is typical of an extradural haematoma. This form of extradural collection is produced by a tear, usually in the middle meningeal artery in the temporal or parietal region. The haematoma generally develops more quickly than the subdural collections because it originates in an arterial bleed. However, the bleeding occurs in the extradural space where the dura is tightly adherent to the vault and haematoma cannot spread easily and collects in this lens-shaped lesion. The history of a brief period of recovery before eventually deteriorating consciousness is very suggestive of this diagnosis. Its appearance on the CT scan is quite specific and is normally considered a neurosurgical emergency.

Scan C shows a smaller, older lesion in another patient.

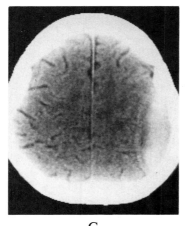

C

Case 8

Female, aged 52 years.

Weakness of right side and fits for 5 years.

Mild right-sided weakness; right homonymous hemianopia.

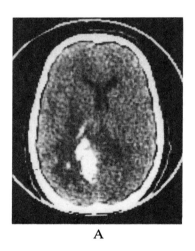

A

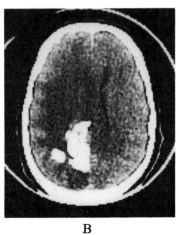

B

Case 8

Calcified tumour (oligodendroglioma)

Scans A and B show irregular high density material throughout the left posterior parietal and occipital lobes, and extending deeply as far as the splenium (scan B), and inferiorly to the left thalamus (scan A). There is a mass effect with midline shift to the right. Density measurements show this to be in the range 110–190 Hounsfield units consistent with calcification. Such calcification may be seen in: low grade tumours; aneurysms (a most unlikely site!) (*see* Case 4); old trauma (there was no history of injury in this case); Sturge-Weber syndrome (*see* Case 9) usually associated with marked local atrophy; AVMs usually showing marked serpiginous enhancement. Because of the latter possibility, contrast medium was given. This showed no change. These features together with the midline shift suggest this is most likely to be a low grade tumour. This degree of calcification suggests an oligodendroglioma—a slow-growing, low grade tumour. Astrocytomas, teratomas and dermoids could look like this but usually show more mixed densities.

(Oligodendrogliomas usually show unimpressive enhancement and are therefore included in this group of high density non-enhancing lesions.)

The visual field disorder is entirely consistent with a lesion in the occipital lobe.

Case 9

Male, aged 27 years.

Long history of focal seizures and right hemiparesis.

Port-wine stain on left side of face.

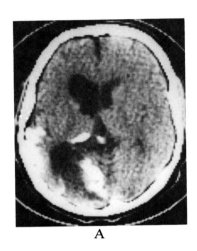

A

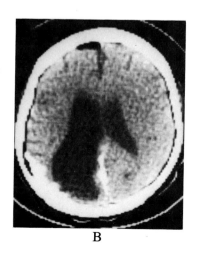

B

Case 9

Sturge–Weber syndrome

Plain scans A and B show focal dilatation of the occipital horn of the left lateral ventricle. There is extensive calcification around the occipital lobe cortex extending along the midline and over the surface of the hemisphere into the parietal area. There was no change after contrast enhancement. The dilatation of the occipital horn is very important as it appears drawn towards the dystrophic calcified gyri on the cortex indicating local atrophy. The history of fits and a facial venous angioma are typical of this condition, where there is an associated but physically separate capillary disorder of the occipital/parietal cortex with atrophy and dystrophic calcification.

Although apparently due to a diffuse capillary angiomatous situation, most of these do not have an obvious vascular malformation in the cortex by the time they are scanned, and enhancement is usually minimal or absent (presumably the result of atrophy). Compare this with Case 8 where the main distinguishing features are the absence of atrophy and non-cortical distribution of the calcification.

Case 10

Female, aged 23 years.

Six month history of right hemiparesis.

No other neurological signs.

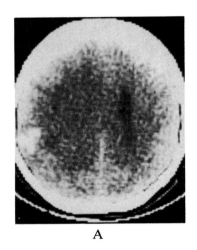

A

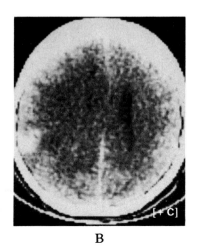

B

Case 10

Calcified astrocytoma

Plain scan A shows a calcified lesion in the high left parietal area close to the vault but separated from it. There is no real change after contrast enhancement (scan B). The ventricles are a little dilated and displaced away from the lesion. The absence of a history of previous injury which could have given rise to a dystrophic calcification in the area makes the diagnosis of a low grade calcified tumour a strong possibility. Many of these have associated low density components (*see* Case 52) but some do not. An AVM should show marked enhancement (*see* Cases 15 and 56). The presence of calcification in a tumour usually indicates a reasonably low grade type such as astrocytoma or oligodendroglioma. Other enhancing calcified tumours are described in other sections. Biopsy confirmed this to be a low grade astrocytoma and it was successfully removed.

Case 11

Female, aged 71 years.

Left nerve deafness. Diminished left Vth sensation.

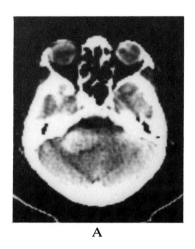

A

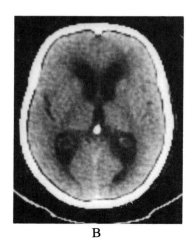

B

Case 11

Calcified and thrombosed aneurysm

Scan A shows a dense and partly calcified mass in the left cerebello-pontine angle. The fourth ventricle is obliterated by pressure and there is resultant hydrocephalus (scan B). Scans after enhancement showed no change. The commonest lesion in the cerebello-pontine angle is an acoustic neuroma, but these invariably show definite enhancement and calcification is unusual. The skull films did not show any enlargement of the internal auditory meatus, another finding which one would expect with an acoustic tumour. Angiography and subsequent surgery showed this to be a largely thrombosed aneurysm of the posterior inferior cerebellar artery. The thrombosis explains why the lesion did not enhance on CT. Giant aneurysms are not uncommon and should always be kept in mind with lesions close to the site of major vessels. Most of them are seen close to the suprasellar cistern (*see* Cases 4, 14 and 70).

Shown below (image C) is the vertebral arteriogram of this patient. The partly thrombosed aneurysm is clearly shown.

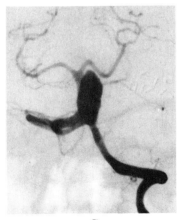

C

Case 12

Female, aged 16 years.

Increasing incoordination and deteriorating consciousness in spina bifida patient with known ventricular shunt.

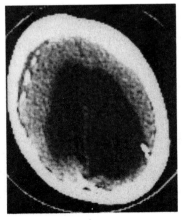

A

Case 12

Calcified subdural haematoma

Plain scan A shows markedly dilated ventricles suggesting a failure of the shunt from blockage or some other cause. A rim of calcification deep to a low density area is seen over the surface of the left hemisphere. This is a chronic subdural haematoma, a not uncommon complication of shunting dilated ventricles, but more usually the result of head injury (*see* Case 28). Some of the haematomas of very long standing calcify.

Calcification this close to the vault may be due to a tumour (Case 10), meningioma or osteoma. The latter is clearly attached to the vault and unlike a meningioma does not enhance. Benign dural calcification may also look like this.

Scan B (another patient) shows calcification over the left parietal area due to a previous bout of meningitis.

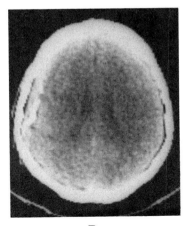

B

47

Case 13

Male, aged 13 years.

Fits for many years, recently increasing in frequency.

Rash on face. Some mental retardation.

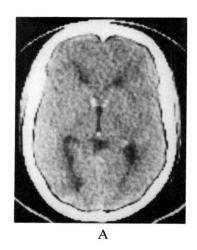

A

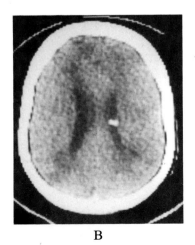

B

Case 13

Tuberous sclerosis

Scans A and B show flecks of calcification in the ependymal wall of the ventricles in several places. This appearance is quite typical of tuberous sclerosis. Some of the tubers may not be calcified and therefore difficult to identify. Some patients may show associated hydrocephalus and a small proportion of patients may develop an astrocytoma. This will show as a bigger lesion and may exhibit enhancement.

The only other conditions likely to produce a similar appearance are toxoplasmosis and cytomegalic inclusion disease (CMID). Both are intracranial infections in infants. Toxoplasmosis tends to show calcifications away from the ventricular system, e.g. in the head of the caudate nucleus. CMID looks like tuberous sclerosis, but the calcification tends to occur in sheets rather than in flecks. Both are much less common than tuberous sclerosis.

Case 14

Male, aged 35 years.

Paresis of right Vth and VIth cranial nerves.

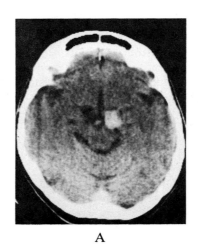

A

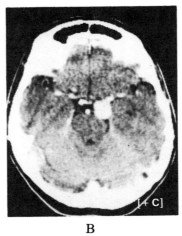

B

Case 14

Aneurysm

Scan A shows a well-circumscribed area of raised density in the right side of the suprasellar cistern. Following contrast enhancement, scan B shows a further increase in density. Its proximity to the vessels of the circle of Willis can be appreciated. On the plain scan some of its densities were in the calcium range.

This lesion is too far lateral to be included in the diagnostic possibilities for pituitary masses (*see* Case 70). A meningioma arising from the dorsum sella or anterior attachments of the tentorium is certainly a possibility (*see* Cases 17, 18, 60). Neuroma of the Vth or VIth cranial nerves could look very like this and produce these symptoms (*see* Case 59). But any lesion with this intense enhancement and particularly close to major vessels must be suspected to be an aneurysm.

This was a giant aneurysm some 3 cm in diameter. Their usual sites of occurrence are shown in Case 4.

Case 15

Female, aged 59 years.

Left hemiparesis (mild) for many years. Recent severe headache, now improved.

Mild weakness of left limbs.

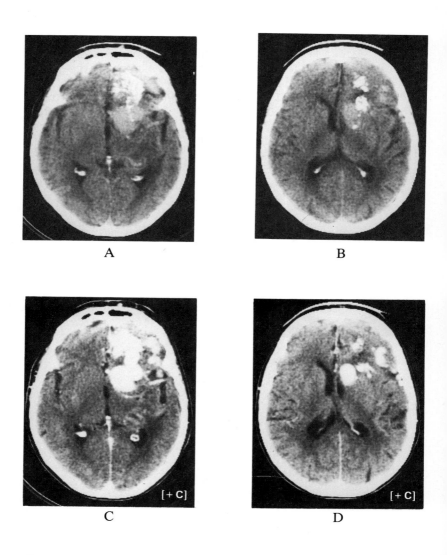

A

B

C

D

Case 15

Arterio-venous malformation (AVM)

Scans A and B show a large lobulated lesion of varying high density in the right hemisphere. In the frontal lobe the density is very high suggesting blood or calcification. This was analysed and shown to be calcification. Behind this are further areas of raised density. Following enhancement (scans C and D) the areas of less raised density show striking enhancement which have a clearcut serpiginous appearance.

These appearances could be due to a tumour, but most calcified tumours tend to be fairly benign and should not enhance to this extent.

This degree and form of enhancement suggest large vascular structures, and in this case these are large dilated veins leading away from an AVM. Other slices showed blood in the ventricular system consistent with the recent story of a bleed (*see* Cases 3 and 56).

Shown below (image E) is an arteriogram demonstrating the highly vascular nature of these congenital lesions with characteristic rapid arterio-venous shunting.

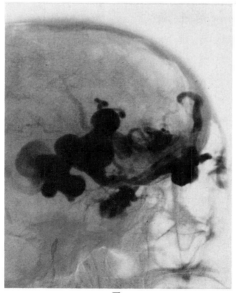

E

Case 16

Female, aged 85 years.

Sudden severe headache and neurological deterioration in a patient with several months' history of progressive dementia and weakness of legs.

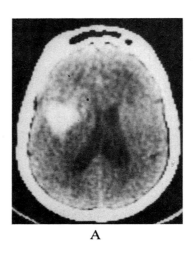

A

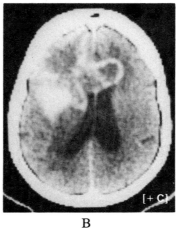

B

Case 16

Acute haemorrhage in corpus callosum glioma

Plain scan A shows a high density area in the left basal nuclei and adjacent sylvian fissure. There is some midline shift to the right and also a vague low density area in front of the ventricles. Because of this latter feature and the absence of a history of injury or hypertension, constrast medium was given. Scan B shows irregular enhancement in front of both ventricles consistent with a malignant glioma in the genu of the corpus callosum. This appearance could also be due to a metastatic deposit. For the appearance of gliomas *see* Cases 44 and 45.

Many intracranial tumours can bleed and most seemingly benign intracranial haemorrhages should be followed up later to see if any other lesion remains after the haemorrhage has cleared (*see* Case 3).

Case 17

Male, aged 52 years.

Seven months' history of headaches and temporal lobe epilepsy.

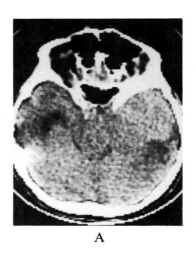

A

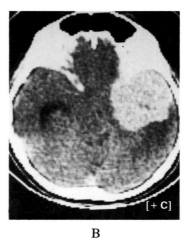

B

Case 17

Meningioma

Scan A shows a dilated temporal horn on the left. On the right side there is a vague area of increased density in the middle cranial fossa. There is a suggestion of some thickening of the greater wing of sphenoid on the right. After contrast enhancement scan B shows dramatic increase in density throughout the lesion. This is well defined and extends up to the sphenoid ridge.

The appearances are typical of a meningioma. These benign tumours arise from the dural coverings of the brain and so are found along the base of the brain, along the falx and tentorium, the petrous ridge, foramen magnum, etc. They are invariably slightly denser than brain on the plain scan and show marked enhancement. They are well defined and about 15 per cent show calcification. Their peripheral position is characteristic and a definitive diagnosis can be made by angiography. Meningiomas in other sites are discussed in Cases 18, 50 and 60.

Female, aged 44 years.

Four month history of right-sided weakness and focal fits.

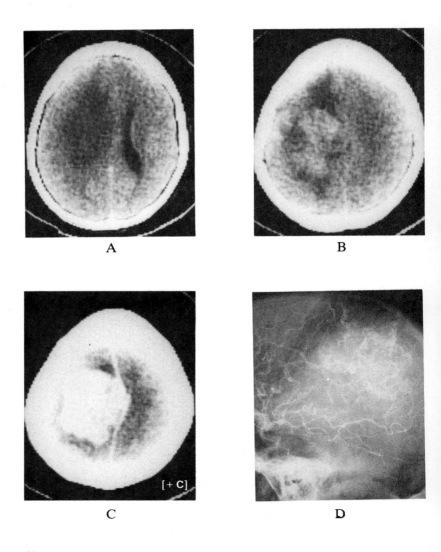

A

B

C [+ C]

D

Case 18

Meningioma

Scan A shows an area of cerebral swelling in the upper left hemi-sphere with compression of the left lateral ventricle and midline shift to the right. Scan B shows a raised density lesion in the left para sagit-tal area close to the vertex. Scan C shows dramatic enhancement in this well-defined lesion which is arising from and distorting the en-hanced falx.

This lesion has all the characteristics of a meningioma (*see* Cases 17, 50, 60), the position being one of the classic sites. An arteriogram (D) confirms the highly vascular nature of these tumours and specific blood supply from branches of the external carotid. This is not an appropriate site for an aneurysm. An AVM and lymphoma would also have to be considered (*see* Cases 15 and 19). Metastasis is a pos-sibility in any enhancing lesion.

Shown below is an unusual form of the lesion. The meningioma is spread over the floor of the middle fossa like a plate: the so-called 'meningioma-en-plaque'. The only evidence for it on Scan E is a vague uptake low in the middle fossa on the right.

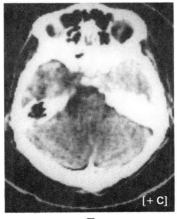

E

Case 19

Female, aged 67 years.

Headache, intellectual loss of 6 months' duration.

Mild dementia. Right hemiparesis.

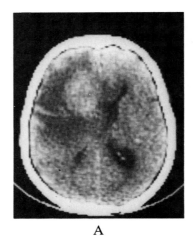

A

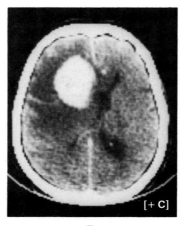

B

Case 19

Primary lymphoma of brain (microglioma)

Plain scan A shows an area of raised density in the depths of the left frontal lobe with deformity of the left frontal horn and midline shift to the right. The lesion is surrounded by a wide band of oedema. Enhanced scan B shows a diffuse strong pattern of enhancement. The lesion did not extend to the skull base. The possibilities include: meningioma (this would be an unusual site away from dura); giant aneurysm (arteriogram advisable); metastatic deposit; arteriovenous malformation; granuloma. An arteriogram was unhelpful and a biopsy showed this to be a lymphoma. Primary lymphoma of the brain (used to be called 'microglioma') is not uncommon and because it responds well to radiotherapy it is a worthwhile diagnosis to make. Its usual appearance is like this and in an appropriate site looks very similar to meningioma. Following therapy, the patient showed the appearance below (scan C enhanced) with dramatic resolution. Enhancement around the edge of the ventricles is now present. This is another feature of this condition and may be its only manifestation. This type can mimic ventriculitis (*see* Case 77).

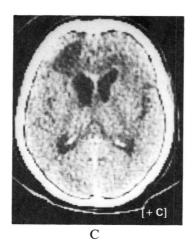

C

Case 20

Male, aged 61 years.

Recent onset of epilepsy.

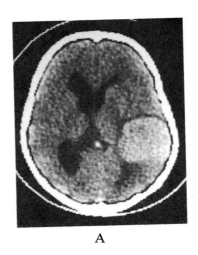

A

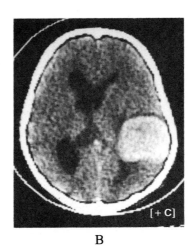

B

Case 20

Metastatic deposit

Scan A shows a well-circumscribed lesion of raised density in the right parietal area. There is some associated mass effect with compression of the right ventricle and dilatation of the left and midline shift to the left. Following contrast enhancement, scan B shows a definite increase in density throughout the lesion.

The appearances could well be due to a meningioma because of its proximity to the vault (Case 17). Lymphoma is also a possibility (Case 19). But angiography failed to reveal any evidence of a meningioma. The patient had a previous history of a malignant melanoma removed from his right thigh 3 years previously and biopsy confirmed that this was a solitary metastatic deposit. Metastases are very common in the brain and can look like practically anything, but they invariably enhance. Melanoma metastases are usually dense like this on the plain scan. (*See also* Cases 46, 51 and 83.)

Case 21

Male, aged 9 years.

Vomiting and headaches for 9 months.

Papilloedema.

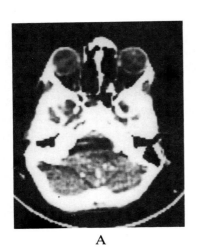

A

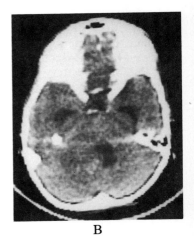

B

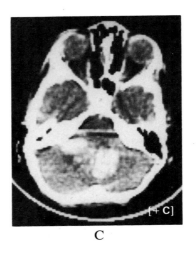

[+C]

C

Case 21

Ependymoma

Scan A shows several areas of high density low in the posterior fossa. Scan B shows dilated temporal horns due to hydrocephalus and the distortion of the fourth ventricle that is causing this. After enhancement scan C shows extensive increased density in the posterior fossa.

This lesion might be an AVM (*see* Case 15), but angiography showed no evidence of this or meningioma. The most likely possibilities here are medulloblastoma or ependymoma. These are the commonest tumours in the posterior fossa in childhood. These conditions are discussed in Cases 61 and 62. Choroid plexus papilloma also has to be considered (*see* Case 24).

Case 22

Female, aged 37 years.

Intermittent severe headache.

Early papilloedema.

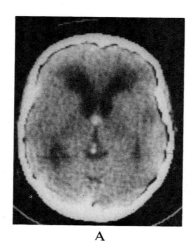

A

Case 22

Colloid cyst

Scan A shows a raised density lesion in the midline related to the third ventricle at the level of the foramina of Munro. The lateral ventricles are dilated. There was some increased density after enhancement. This appearance is highly suggestive of a colloid cyst. The site and density are typical. Some of these lesions however can be difficult to see as they are not always of raised density, and the hydrocephalus may be intermittent due to a ball-valve type of action. Scan B shows a large lesion that is almost as dense as brain.

Scan C shows a further example of a colloid cyst in which the lesion itself is not seen but can be inferred from the obliterated third ventricle.

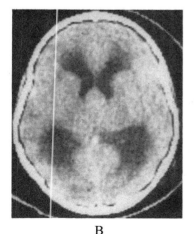

B

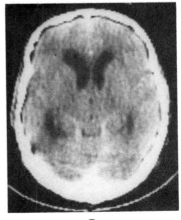

C

Case 23

Male, aged 42 years.

Intermittent severe headaches.

Papilloedema.

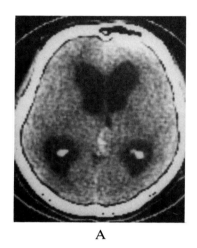

A

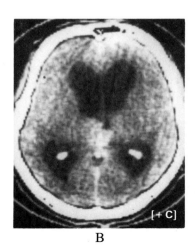

B

Case 23

Pinealoma

Scan A shows an area of pineal calcification that is larger than usual and is associated with a soft tissue mass around it and some dilatation of the ventricles. Contrast-enhanced scan B shows extensive enhancement in the uncalcified part of the mass. The appearance and position of the lesion are typical of pinealoma, and hydrocephalus is often associated. The appearances may be mimicked by meningiomas arising from the tentorium, or by gliomas in the posterior part of the third ventricle.

Case 24

Female, aged 32 years.

Intermittent severe headaches and vomiting.

Papilloedema, vertigo.

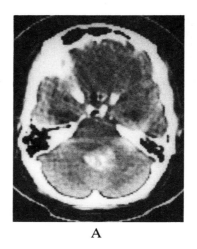

A

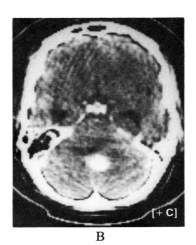

B

Case 24

Choroid plexus papilloma

Scan A shows a high density lesion occupying the fourth ventricle. Some of its density was found to be in the range of calcium. After enhancement scan B shows marked enhancement. The temporal horns are dilated due to hydrocephalus. The differential diagnosis includes choroid plexus papilloma (a tumour of the choroid associated with excess CSF production, hence the hydrocephalus) and ependymoma (commonly found in the fourth ventricle looks just like this, *see* Case 21). Medulloblastoma and intraventricular meningioma would also be difficult to distinguish. Choroid plexus papilloma may also be found elsewhere in the ventricles and tends to spread along the CSF spaces.

Scan C (same patient) shows spread in the CSF to the suprasellar cistern 2 years later.

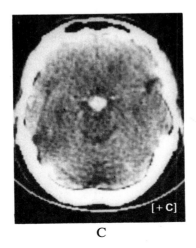

C

71

Case 25

Female, aged 18 years.

Headaches and confusion for 2 years. Vomiting. Some intermittent weakness of limbs.

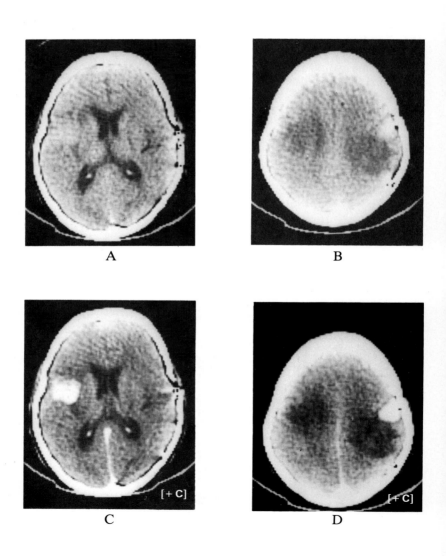

A

B

C

D

Case 25

Cerebral tuberculosis

Scans A and B show vague areas of high density in both hemispheres. There is also some low density. There has been a previous right craniotomy. After contrast, scans C and D show dramatic enhancement in the previously raised density areas. These changes are not specific and a wide range of possible diagnoses have to be considered including multiple metastases, AVMs, meningiomas, etc. At a previous craniotomy a tuberculoma was removed. This condition is still very common in certain parts of the world and it should be kept in mind in any enhancing lesion. It often mimics a malignant glioma.

Case 26

Female, aged 29 years.

Long history of epilepsy.

Some weakness of right limbs.

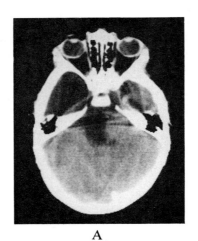

A

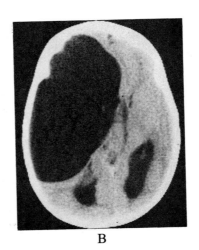

B

Case 26

Arachnoid cyst

Scan A shows a low density (fluid) area in the left temporal region with expansion of the bony middle fossa and extension of the lesion into the posterior fossa. Scan B shows the same lesion higher up, with midline shift. The ventricles are mildly dilated. The site and appearances are typical of a congenital arachnoid cyst. It is unusual to see one this size (but *see also* scan C). The expansion of the middle fossa is typical and is consistent with a long history. The sylvian fissure is a common site (*see below* scan D). Arachnoid cysts are also found in the posterior fossa (not to be confused with a large cisterna magna which unlike the cyst is midline). Other possibilities for this lesion are a grossly dilated temporal horn or porencephalic cyst, but there was nothing to suggest a ventricular communication. This could be confirmed with dye in the CSF.

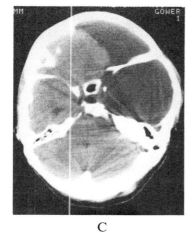

C

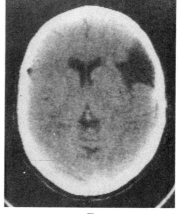

D

Case 27

Male, aged 37 years.

Epilepsy for 7 years. Vague headaches.

Some weakness of right limbs since childhood.

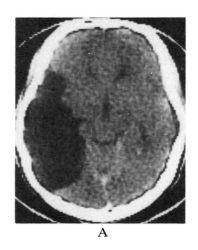

A

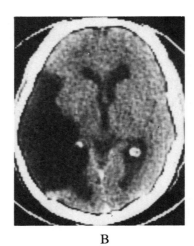

B

Case 27

Porencephalic cyst

Scan A shows a low density area in the left temporal region with some thinning of the overlying bone. Scan B shows that it is continuous with the left trigone area and producing very little mass effect. Its communication with the ventricle was confirmed by intraventricular contrast medium. Its general appearance is similar to the arachnoid cyst in Case 26, but continuity with the ventricle is characteristic of porencephaly. Porencephalic cysts may be congenital or acquired from trauma, surgery, etc.

Scan C shows a further example communicating with the superior aspect of the lateral ventricle.

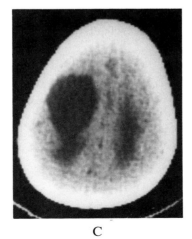

C

Case 28

Female, aged 75 years.

Ten-week history of gradual onset of confusion.

Mild left hemiparesis.

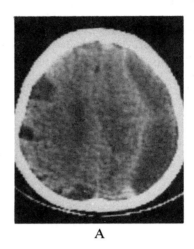

A

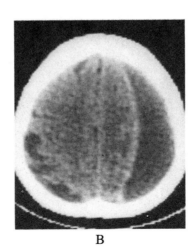

B

Case 28

Chronic subdural haematoma

Scans A and B show a well-defined low density lesion overlying the surface of the upper right cerebral hemisphere. There is some shift of midline structures to the left and atrophy in the left hemisphere. The density of this lesion suggests fluid, but it is not as low in density as CSF. The way in which it lies over the upper hemisphere is entirely consistent with a chronic subdural haematoma.

This lesion usually occurs as a delayed result of head injury. The patient is often elderly and a history of injury may not be forthcoming. The story may contain elements of dementia, headache and slowly progressive neurological defect. The initial head injury produces a shallow acute subdural haematoma (*see* Case 6) which goes unnoticed. As the weeks pass the blood becomes organized and a capsule is formed and an osmotic pressure is set up drawing low density fluid into the old haematoma, hence the low density. The lesion may take weeks or months to reach the stage shown here and from an initial high density stage passes through a phase where the haematoma is the same density as brain (isodense) before reaching this low density phase. (*See also* Case 36.)

Case 29

Female, aged 30 years.

One-year history of headache and change of personality.

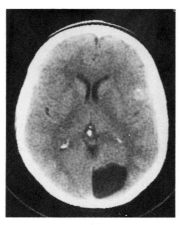

A

Case 29

Astrocytoma (cystic)

Scan A shows a well-defined low density lesion in the right occipital lobe. Contrast enhancement showed no change. There is some mass effect with the right trigone displaced away from the lesion. The sharp margin suggests a cyst and the density is similar to CSF. The mass effect is against infarction (*see* Cases 30 and 32).) Biopsy showed a cystic astrocytoma. Cystic astrocytomas represent the more benign end of the scale of gliomas. Other features suggesting benign characteristics include calcification (*see* Case 10). The presence of enhancement suggests a more malignant astrocytoma (*see* Case 52) and florid enhancement with necrosis is seen in the highly malignant grade of glioma (*see* Cases 44 and 45).

Scan B shows an ill-defined non-cystic astrocytoma which also did not enhance and was of low grade. A lesion of this appearance is indistinguishable from local cerebral oedema due to some other process, and presents considerable difficulty in diagnosis (*see* Cases 33 and 34).

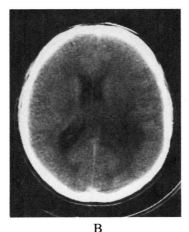

B

Case 30

Male, aged 63 years.

Four-month history of hemianopia of sudden onset.

Left visual field loss.

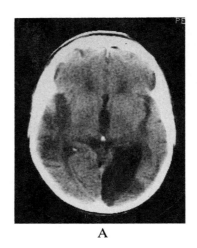

A

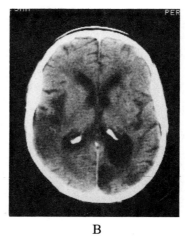

B

Case 30

Old infarct

Scans A and B show a low density area in the right occipital pole. On scan B it can be seen that the lesion has a faint line of demarcation from the ventricle which is dilated in that area. There is no evidence of a mass effect and there was no change after contrast enhancement. A further lesion is present in the middle cerebral area on the left.

The appearances are typical of an old infarct in the territory of the posterior cerebral artery. The distribution of the lesion within the territory supplied by a vessel, the absence of a mass effect and the presence of an element of atrophy as indicated by the focal dilatation of the ventricle (*see* Case 35), all point to an old infarct rather than a tumour or porencephalic cyst.

Infarcts tend to occur in the whole or part of the territory of a major vessel such as the anterior cerebral, middle cerebral or posterior cerebral. Their areas of supply are shown in diagram C. Scan D shows an old infarct involving the middle and posterior cerebral artery territories on the left with atrophy in this area causing the left ventricle to enlarge and be displaced towards this side. (*See* Cases 35 and 80.)

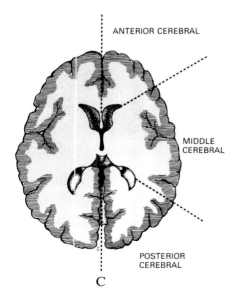

ANTERIOR CEREBRAL

MIDDLE CEREBRAL

POSTERIOR CEREBRAL

C

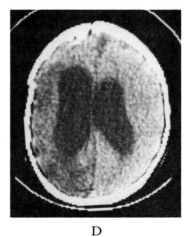

D

Male, aged 29 years.

History of fits and personality disorder since severe head injury 5 years previously.

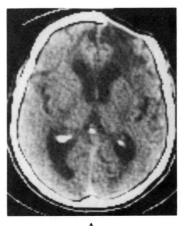

A

Case 31

Brain 'softening' following trauma/surgery

Scan A shows a defect in the vault in the right frontal region. Deep to this is an ill-defined low density area in the right frontal lobe with some focal dilatation of the frontal horn of the right lateral ventricle. There was no change after contrast enhancement.

The history of head injury and bony defect in the frontal area are crucial and confirm the suspicion that the patient suffered severe contusion to the frontal lobe (due to a depressed fracture) and has ended up with an atrophic frontal lobe. A similar process may be seen after surgery, radiation therapy (*see* scan B below), haematomas, infarcts, etc. In many instances the process is called 'softening' but in some cases an actual cyst is formed.

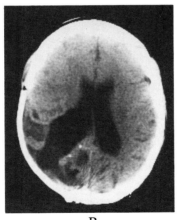

B

Case 32

Male, aged 50 years.

Sudden onset of collapse and left-sided weakness 5 days ago, steadily improving.

Moderate residual left hemiparesis.

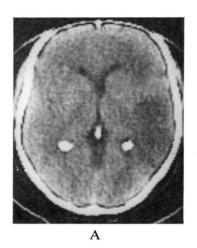

A

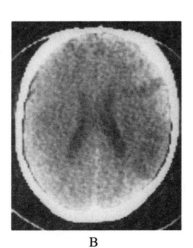

B

Case 32

Recent infarct

Scans A and B show a low density area without mass effect in the territory defined by the right middle cerebral artery. The deepest part and some of the area anteriorly is spared. There was no change after contrast. The position of the lesion and its demarcation and absence of mass effect are typical of an infarct. Focal oedema due to trauma or encephalitis is invariably associated with some mass effect. Many recent infarcts show enhancement due to collateral blood flow (*see* Cases 41 and 42) but some do not, such as the present case. Sparing of parts of the vessel's territory is also common. As infarcts age there is some cyst formation and atrophy and the infarcted area becomes less dense (*see* Case 30).

Case 33

Female, aged 19 years.

Sudden onset (over 2 hours) of headache, dysphasia and confusion. Taking oral contraceptive.

Expressive dysphasia, severe confusion.

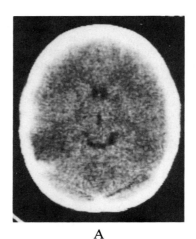

A

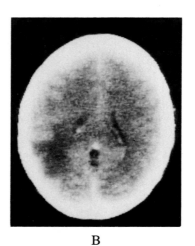

B

Case 33

Venous infarction

Scan A shows an ill-defined low density area in the left posterior temporal area. Scan B shows the same pathology at a higher level. There was no contrast enhancement. These changes are quite non-specific, but the rapid onset suggested infarction or encephalitis. This appearance is due to infarction resulting from venous occlusion, usually in cortical veins and/or venous sinuses. This is not an uncommon occurrence in young females on oral contraceptives, or in the post-partum period.

Confirmation can be achieved by angiography to show occluded veins, or, as in this case, an isotope study of the venous sinuses (image C) which shows a normal sigmoid sinus on the right and occlusion on the left.

Thrombosis of the superior sagittal sinus is demonstrated in Case 81.

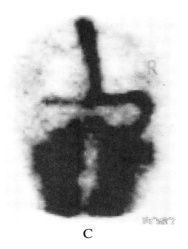

C

Case 34

Female, aged 31 years.

One-week history of increasing confusion and now semi-comatose.

Low grade fever.

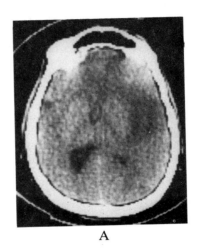

A

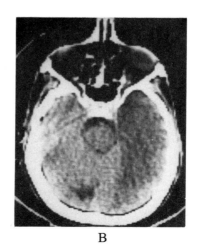

B

Case 34

Encephalitis

Scan A shows small ventricles (compressed) which are displaced to the left by an ill-defined low density area in the right temporal lobe. There was no change after contrast enhancement. Three days later scan B shows the lesion has spread throughout the right temporal lobe. The appearance is that of focal cerebral oedema (*see* Case 37). The history suggests some process other than tumour and there was no history or signs of a head injury. The position of the lesion and the clinical signs suggest encephalitis. This condition often starts in the insula and may spread into the temporal and frontal lobes. The main differential diagnosis would be cerebral abscess, but this shows characteristic enhancement (*see* Case 47). Clinically acute meningitis is very similar but CT scan would only show hydrocephalus if anything. Venous infarction can also look like this (*see* Case 33). Arterial infarction is not usually associated with shift.

Many cases of encephalitis will show a normal scan especially during the first 4 or 5 days of the illness. Some cases show non-specific patterns of enhancement.

Case 35

Male, aged 50 years.

Left hemiparesis and mental handicap since birth, now deteriorating.

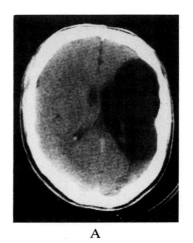

A

Case 35

Birth infarct

Scan A shows a well-defined low density area in the right temporal area with slight midline shift towards the lesion and dilatation of the right ventricle indicating associated atrophy. The anterior extent of the lesion is limited by the margin of the middle cerebral artery territory (*see* Case 30) and posteriorly it also does not extend beyond this territory. This suggests an infarct and the atrophy indicates that it is of long standing. (There is also compensatory thickening of the vault on this side to support this.)

Difficult delivery of an infant is not uncommonly associated with injuries to the head and neck and an infarct such as this may result. This lesion is probably cystic, a not uncommon finding in old severe infarcts. It is separate from the ventricle (*see* Case 27).

Case 36

Female, aged 63 years.

Three-week history of headache and confusion following minor head injury.

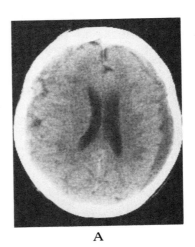

A

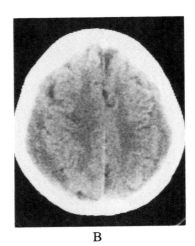

B

Case 36

Chronic subdural haematoma (isodense and bilateral)

Scan A shows a shallow low density collection over the right hemisphere. Its configuration is similar to that of Case 28. The ventricles are mildly displaced towards this side which may be due to atrophy on the right (for which there is no evidence such as local ventricular dilatation) or a mass effect on the left. Scan B taken at a higher level shows a further low density collection over the upper left hemisphere. This one is not so easy to see because the subdural haematoma is sufficiently old to have reached the isodense phase (*see* Case 28). The collection on the right is more mature and therefore less dense. It is sometimes practically impossible to identify an isodense subdural haematoma with certainty when its density is equivalent to brain (contrast enhancement may help to show its margin). In this situation the only evidence for its presence may be midline shift and compression of the ventricle. Such a case is shown in scan C. A subdural haematoma was present on the left and can be shown by arteriography or isotope brain scanning.

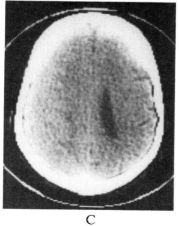

C

Male, aged 22 years.

Three-day history of increasing intellectual impairment and head-ache.

Mild left-sided weakness, now semi-comatose.

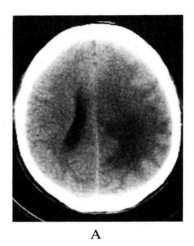

A

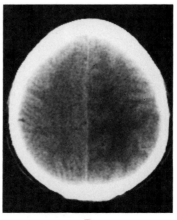

B

Case 37

Cerebral oedema

Scan A shows an extensive ill-defined low density area in the right hemisphere. The right ventricle is obliterated by compression and there is some shift of midline structures (corpus callosum) to the left. Scan B shows the same process at a higher level. It can readily be seen that the margins of this low density area are serrated; this pattern is due to the process being confined to the white matter, the grey matter being relatively uninvolved. There was no change after contrast enhancement.

These changes reflect focal swelling of the brain or cerebral oedema. This can be caused by a wide variety of things including trauma, infections such as abscesses and encephalitis, tumours, metastases, surgery, infarcts (especially venous) and a variety of toxic conditions. Many of these will show enhancement. The history will often be vital and factors such as fever, a recent head injury, etc., will point to the correct diagnosis. A longer history may indicate a low grade glioma (*see* Case 29).

Case 38

Male, aged 5 years.

Six-week history of intellectual loss and generalized weakness.

Widespread neurological deficits.

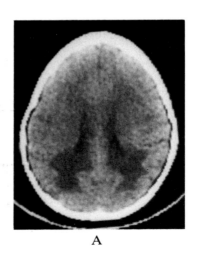

A

Case 38

Adreno-leucodystrophy

Scan A shows symmetrical low density areas in both occipital lobes adjacent to the ventricles. There was no change after contrast enhancement. This looks like symmetrical cerebral oedema but there was no history of head injury. Some tumours of the posterior part of the corpus callosum can produce this sort of pattern but should show midline involvement which is obviously not present. The age and sex of the patient coupled with the symmetrical and posteriorly placed lesions are very suggestive of adreno-leucodystrophy. This is a rare progressive brain degeneration of unknown cause associated with adrenal gland dysfunction and usually occurs in young boys. The condition is gradually progressive and scan B shows the same patient 16 months later when there is widespread brain degeneration.

A similar symmetrical degeneration due to leucodystrophy (leuco-encephalopathy) can be seen in adults (usually frontal lobes) in some other rare disorders.

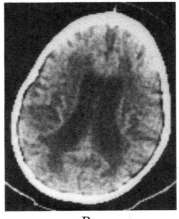

B

Case 39

Male, aged 71 years.

Intermittent dementia deteriorating over 3½ months.

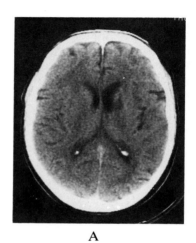

A

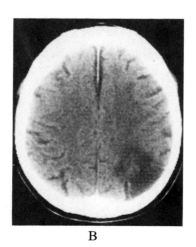

B

Case 39

Multiple infarcts

Scan A shows a well-defined low density area in the right caudate nucleus. The adjacent right frontal horn of the lateral ventricle is mildly dilated suggesting associated atrophy. Scan B shows a wedge-shaped area of low density in the right parietal area posteriorly. Both these lesions have characteristics suggesting infarcts (*see* Case 30). There was no change after contrast enhancement. Other possibilities include multiple metastases (these invariably show some enhancement) and multiple sclerosis. This latter condition would be unusual at this age and lesions are usually paraventricular and rarely become as obvious as these.

Scan C shows a further example with characteristic wedge-shaped lesions in the left anterior cerebral territory and the posterior part of the middle cerebral territory.

Multiple infarcts are a common finding in demented patients and a major differential of Alzheimer's disease (*see* Case 78).

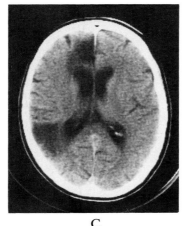

C

Case 40

Male, aged 73 years.

Lifetime history of paranoid delusion and self-neglect.

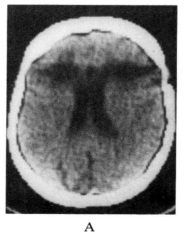

A

Case 40

Previous leucotomy

Scan A shows symmetrical transverse bands across both frontal lobes. There is also some irregularity of the skull vault on the right, overlying the lesion.

These lesions do not follow any known pathological process. They are in fact the result of bilateral surgery. The operation is known as 'leucotomy' and produced a partial cutting across the frontal lobes. It was designed to relieve severe long-standing psychiatric disorders. It is now rarely performed and was done more than 20 years ago on this patient.

Female, aged 57 years.

Sudden onset of left-sided weakness 6 days previously.

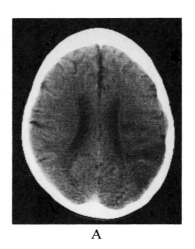

A

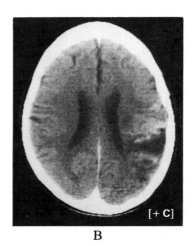

[+ C]

B

Case 41

Acute infarction (middle cerebral artery)

Scan A shows a low density area lateral to the right trigone. This is limited posteriorly by the margin of the middle cerebral artery territory (*see* Case 30). The lesion is not causing midline shift or compression of the trigone. Scan B shows fine enhancement along the margins of the lesion.

These appearances are due to a recent infarct in the posterior half of the middle cerebral artery territory. The position of the lesion is typical. Absence of a mass effect is also usual with infarcts unless they are massive or associated with haemorrhage. This pattern of enhancement is quite common in recent infarcts and takes up to 24–48 hours to appear; it is due to establishment of a collateral circulation along the edges of the infarcted area. The enhancement is often in the form of finger-like processes passing into the area from the outer margin as shown in another case (*see below* scan C). Over a period of weeks this enhancement disappears.

The differential diagnosis of acute infarction is given in Case 42.

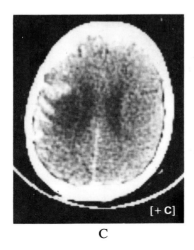

C

Case 42

Female, aged 51 years.

Sudden onset of left hemiparesis 4 days previously.

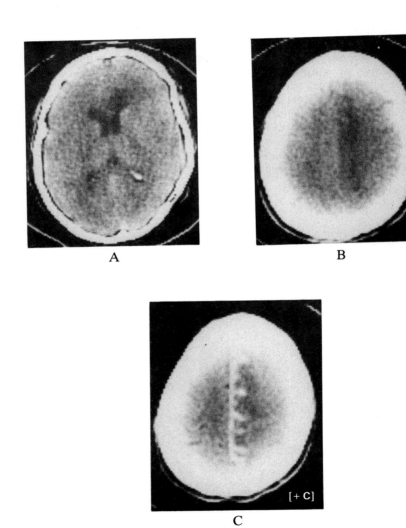

A

B

[+ C]

C

Case 42

Acute infarction (anterior cerebral artery)

Scan A shows a low density lesion to the right of the midline anterior to the frontal horn of the right lateral ventricle. Scan B shows the same lesion running alongside the midline in the upper part of the hemisphere. Scan C shows short finger-like areas of enhancement entering the lesion from its medial margin. This is the enhancement pattern of an infarct and the distribution of the lesion represents part of the territory of the anterior cerebral artery (calloso-marginal artery) which, apart from occupying the anterior wedge of the diagram shown in Case 30, also supplies this strip along the top of the brain.

Many infarcts show enhancement in the early stages but it fades with time. This feature helps to differentiate it from tumours. The pattern of enhancement is usually quite different and the absence of mass effect and the geographical distribution are also important signs. Other enhancing lesions with which infarction may be confused are covered in the ensuing Cases 43-49. Enhancement may also be seen in encephalitis.

Case 43

Female, aged 33 years.

Ten-day history of visual loss and headache.

Fever, right homonymous hemianopia.

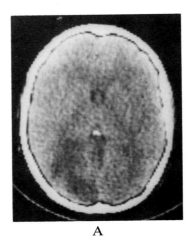

A

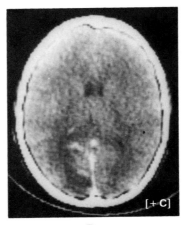

B

Case 43

Septic infarction

Scan A shows a low density area in the left occipital pole (hence the visual field defect). Scan B shows early finger-like enhancement along the posterior and medial margins of the lesion. The appearance of the lesion at this stage is consistent with an infarct in the posterior cerebral territory. But 2 weeks later scan C shows a ring-like area of enhancement posteriorly suggesting an early abscess (*see* Case 47).

The sequence of events and the fever point to a septic infarction. This is due to an infected embolus from septicaemia. Arteriography may show small peripheral mycotic aneurysms which are diagnostic.

These lesions are uncommon and the differential diagnosis must include abscess, glioma and metastases. The history of fever, rapid onset and evidence of infection should suggest this diagnosis.

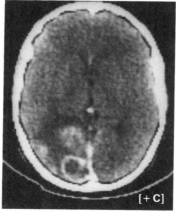

[+ C] 2 weeks later

C

Case 44

Male, aged 35 years.

Five-month history of visual problems, headaches and personality change.

Papilloedema. Left homonymous hemianopia. Some left-sided weakness.

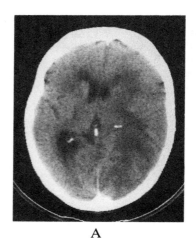

A

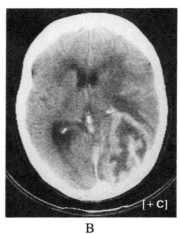

B

Case 44

Malignant glioma

Scan A shows a low density area in the right occipito-parietal area with midline shift to the left and marked forward displacement of the trigone and the choroid plexus on the right. The trigone is virtually obliterated by pressure. After contrast enhancement scan B shows striking irregular enhancement. Much of this is around the edge of the lesion and varies in thickness. Most of the centre of the lesion lies partly in the territory of both middle and posterior cerebral arteries and exhibits a substantial mass effect. These features and the pattern of enhancement are quite unlike an infarct (*see* Case 42). Abscesses invariably show ring-like enhancement (*see* Case 47). The main differentials for this lesion are malignant glioma and a solitary metastasis. These can be very difficult to differentiate but a search elsewhere may reveal a primary or other secondaries. Metastases will be more likely in older patients.

Further details on malignant gliomas are found in Case 45. Shown below in scan C is another malignant glioma in the genu of the corpus callosum where the lesion extends into both frontal lobes.

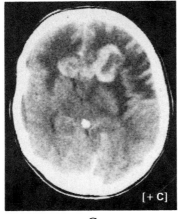

C

111

Case 45

Female, aged 14 years.

Three-month history of headaches.

Papilloedema.

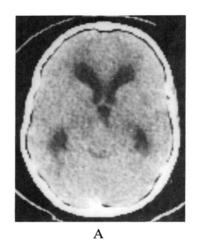

A

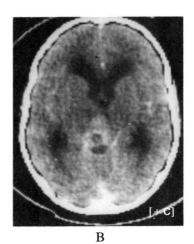

B

Case 45

Malignant glioma

Scan A shows dilatation of the lateral and third ventricles. The posterior end of the third ventricle is narrowed and a vague area of raised density can be seen just to the left of the narrowed segment. Scan B shows enhancement in this area and at the back of the third ventricle. This lesion could be a glioma, or a tumour of the pineal gland but the latter invariably shows marked calcification and enlargement of the gland (*see* Case 23). A biopsy confirmed the presence of a glioma. Surgery was not undertaken as the lesion was considered to be too deep, and radiation therapy was given and the ventricles shunted. Scan C taken 9 months later shows a massive lesion with striking enhancement. The ventricles have dilated further despite the presence of a shunt.

Malignant glioma is the most florid form of the glioma tumours. It is rapidly invasive and shows dramatic enhancement. The less malignant forms are low grade astrocytoma (Case 29) and malignant astrocytoma (Case 52).

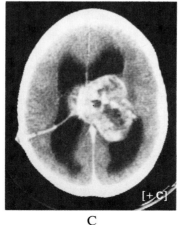

C

Case 46

Male, aged 67 years.

Three-week history of focal fits and headaches.

Papilloedema, moderate left-sided weakness.

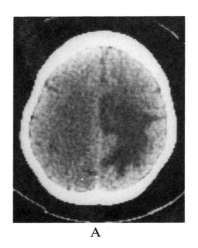

A

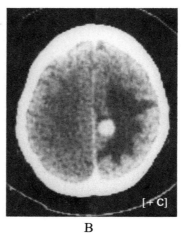

B

Case 46

Metastasis

Scan A shows an area of oedema in the upper right hemisphere. Following enhancement (scan B) there is dense uptake of dye. The lesion could represent a small meningioma arising from the falx but it is in fact a metastasis. Metastases of course are often multiple (*see* Case 83) but the solitary lesions frequently mimic gliomas. Some lesions show high density on the plain scan and so mimic meningioma or lymphoma (*see* Case 20).

The common sources of metastatic deposits in the brain include tumours of bronchus, breast and kidney.

Scan C below, shows another metastatic lesion in the left occipital pole (compare with Case 44).

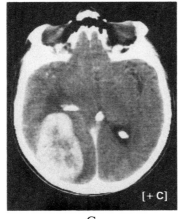

C

Female, aged 50 years.

Nine-day history of fever, headache, confusion.

Semi-comatose, active middle ear infection.

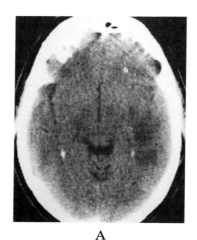

A

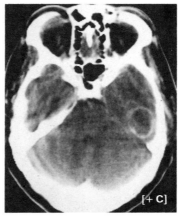

[+ C]

B

Case 47

Cerebral abscess

Scan A shows an extensive area of low density in the right temporal lobe. This is showing some mass effect. After contrast enhancement scan B shows a regular thin-walled ring of enhancement around a fluid centre. The appearances are almost diagnostic of a cerebral abscess. Gliomas can enhance like this but the ring is almost always of varying thickness and irregular in outline (*see* Case 44). Metastases may also be difficult to differentiate but an abscess usually has a shorter history and associated fever.

Many abscesses are associated with a focus of infection such as mastoiditis or sinusitis. They can occur in any part of the brain and may be multiple (*see* Case 85). Scan C shows an example with a ring of enhancement in a frontal abscess. The abscess ring is usually very close to a circle in outline.

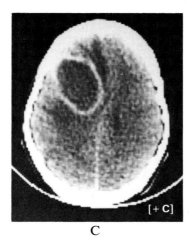

C

Case 48

Male, aged 21 years.

Four-day history of fever and headache.

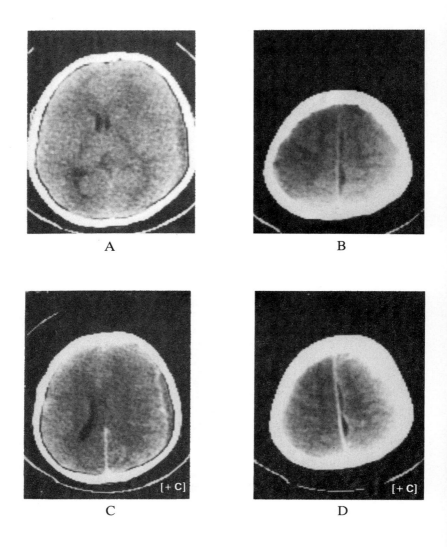

A

B

C

D

Case 48

Subdural abscess

Scan A shows a shallow low density area over the upper right hemisphere similar to a chronic subdural haematoma. Scan B shows a smaller similar lesion adjacent to the falx on the same side. Scans C and D show these areas after contrast enhancement. The margin of these lesions adjacent to the brain is seen to enhance. This appearance may be the only way of delineating a haematoma that is isodense with brain. In this case the lesion is an abscess.

A subdural abscess arises in the subdural space and has similar characteristics to other subdural collections. Easily missed because such abscesses are often small, they invariably show enhancement, and this feature together with the presence of fever should raise the question of a subdural abscess.

Case 49

Male, aged 67 years.

Speech difficulty of sudden onset.

Marked dysphasia.

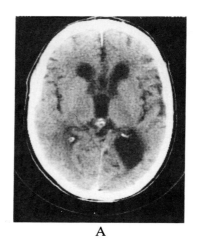

A

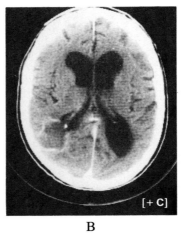

[+ C]

B

Case 49

Enhancing haematoma cavity

Scan A shows dilated ventricles due to atrophy. There is some compression of the posterior part of the left ventricle by a vague low density area just lateral to it. After contrast enhancement scan B shows enhancement around the margin of the lesion.

The lesion crosses the margins of the vascular territories and is unlikely therefore to be an infarct. An abscess would usually have more oedema surrounding the lesion. A glioma or metastasis could look like this but the sudden onset gives the answer. Scan C shows the same patient on admission (10 days before scans A and B). This earlier scan shows a fresh haemorrhage in this site. Many haematomas resorb to leave a cystic area and the margins of these may enhance. This possibility should always be kept in mind for such appearances and an unnecessary biopsy may be avoided by serial scanning.

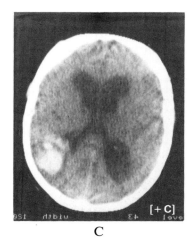

C

Case 50

Male, aged 41 years.

Headaches and inability to smell for 3 years.

Papilloedema.

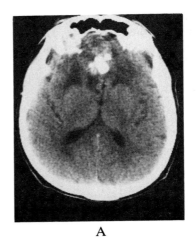

A

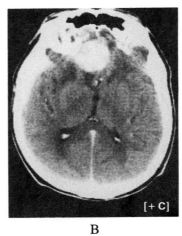

[+ C]

B

Case 50

Meningioma

Scan A shows a lesion with both high and low density adjacent to the skull base in the midline below the frontal lobes. The high density represents calcification. Scan B shows prominent enhancement throughout the lesion.

These characteristics and its position in the olfactory groove are consistent with this being a meningioma (*see* Case 17). Other alternatives to be considered include craniopharyngioma (Case 68) and aneurysm (Case 70). These can be excluded by arteriography.

Male, aged 73 years.

Rapid development of right hemiplegia.

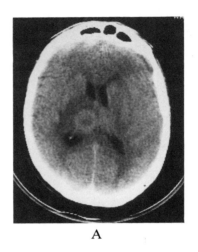

A

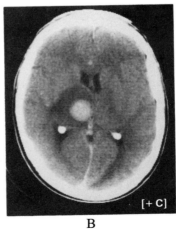

[+ C]

B

Case 51

Metastasis

Scan A shows a lesion of mixed densities in the left thalamic area, with evidence of mass effect. Scan B shows increase in density after contrast enhancement. The appearance could be due to glioma of moderate grade or a metastatic deposit. An AVM could also look like this but there is too much surrounding oedema and the lesion is too regular in appearance. The low density in an AVM is due to focal atrophy (*see* Case 56). A hamartoma is a major possibility in any lesion of mixed density (*see* Case 57). Careful scrutiny of this patient's chest X-ray revealed several faint rounded lesions confirming the suspicion of metastatic disease.

Differentiation between glioma and metastatic disease is often impossible on the CT scan appearances alone in a single lesion, and biopsy is often necessary.

Male, aged 24 years.

Three-year history of increasing weakness of left limbs.

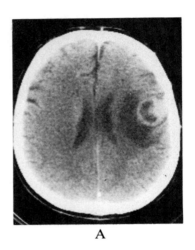

A

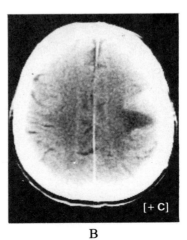

[+ C]

B

Case 52

Malignant astrocytoma

Scan A shows a low density area in the right parietal area associated with a high density area due to calcification. There is some compression and displacement of the right ventricle. Scan B is at a slightly higher level and shows a larger area of enhancement.

This lesion represents a medium grade glioma, the so-called 'malignant astrocytoma'. For a more malignant grade of glioma, *see* Cases 44, 45 and 53. The benign gliomatous tumours are shown in Cases 10 and 29.

Case 53

Male, aged 47 years.

Two-month history of headache and vertigo.

Papilloedema, right-sided weakness.

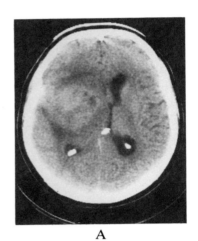

A

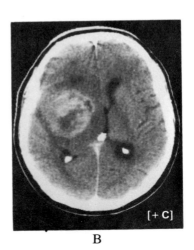

B

Case 53

Malignant glioma

Scan A shows a lesion of high and low densities in the region of the basal nuclei on the left. This is producing a considerable mass effect with compression of the left ventricle and midline shift to the right. Following contrast enhancement scan B shows dramatic and irregular uptake of dye. The appearances would do for a high grade glioma or a metastasis. Biopsy proved this to be a malignant glioma. These lesions may also be wholly of low density before enhancement (*see* Case 44). The centre of this lesion does not enhance due to the presence of necrotic material.

In this case the raised density area on the plain scan may be due to areas of haemorrhage—a common occurrence in this highly malignant lesion (*see* Case 16).

Case 54

Female, aged 75 years.

Sudden onset of visual problems 10 days earlier.

Left homonymous hemianopia.

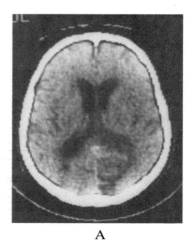

A

Case 54

Haemorrhagic infarct

Scan A shows a low density area in the right occipital lobe. This lesion shows some areas of higher density. There was no change after contrast.

The configuration of this lesion is suggestive of an infarct in the territory of the posterior cerebral artery (*see* Case 30) and indeed this is an infarct, but the areas of higher density are due to a coexisting haemorrhage—a not uncommon variation of the ordinary infarct. This condition should be suspected in any lesion that has all the appearances of an infarct but significant amounts of high density content.

Case 55

Female, aged 70 years.

Three-month history of unsteadiness, confusion.

Mild left-sided weakness.

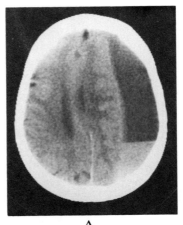

A

Case 55

Mixed density subdural haematoma

Scan A shows a lens-shaped collection overlying the right cerebral hemisphere. This is mostly low density but posteriorly it shows a sediment of high density material. The ventricles are displaced away from this side and compressed. No definite history of injury was forthcoming.

The appearances are those of a chronic subdural haematoma shortly after the isodense phase, when the altered blood products have been able to settle out from the less dense fluid that is continually being drawn into the haematoma. For further details *see* Case 28.

Scan B shows another example of a traumatic lesion of mixed density with a focal area of oedema in which there is an intracortical haemorrhage (right frontal lobe). This has produced ventricular compression and there is probably also a small acute extradural haematoma on the left.

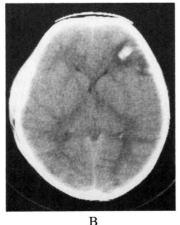

B

Case 56

Male, aged 18 years.

Five-year history of focal epilepsy.

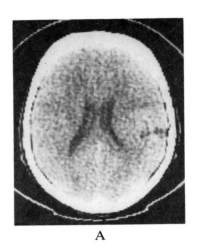

A

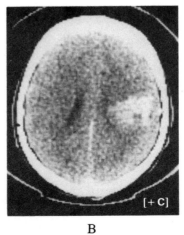

B

Case 56

Arterio-venous malformation (AVM)

Scan A shows an area of high and low density in the right parietal region. There is mild associated compression of the right ventricle. There is quite marked enhancement after contrast medium (scan B).

This lesion could be a medium grade glioma or an AVM (*see* Case 15). Many AVMs show areas of low density due to associated atrophy as in this case (confirmed by arteriography). The appearances are unlike a metastasis where the low density area is wider and less well defined.

Case 57

Male, aged 12 years.

Headaches, vomiting for 4 months.

Papilloedema.

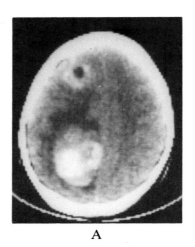

A

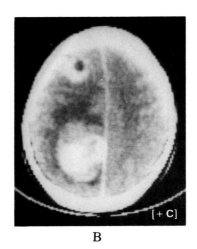

B

Case 57

Hamartoma

Scan A shows areas of raised density (calcification) surrounded by areas of lower density. The most anterior lesion shows a discrete area of very low density (found on measurement to be fat). Scan B shows enhancement in these lesions.

The appearances are non-specific and could be found in a variety of tumours, granulomas, etc. The presence of calcification and fat together however suggests a developmental tumour or hamartoma. Such tumours contain several cell lines hence the variety of tissue densities. They are often quite vascular, hence the enhancement. This diagnosis was confirmed by biopsy.

Case 58

Male, aged 56 years.

Vertigo, tinnitus (right ear) for 7 months.

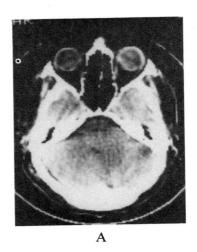

A

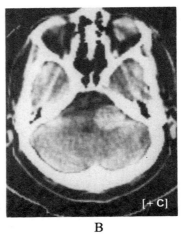

B

Case 58

Acoustic neuroma

Scan A shows some shift of the fourth ventricle to the left. It is not possible to discern any definite abnormality in the cerebellar hemispheres. Scan B shows a well-circumscribed lesion in the right cerebello-pontine angle with prominent enhancement.

The most likely diagnosis here is an acoustic tumour. This lesion is fairly common and is a benign tumour of the eighth cranial nerve. It lies in the cerebello-pontine angle at the orifice of the internal auditory meatus which is usually widened. Many are not visible on the plain scan, and if the story is suggestive then contrast enhancement should be given as they almost always enhance. Some lesions may be of lower or higher density than adjacent brain. Many of them are small and require special techniques for their demonstration. Hydrocephalus is also a common finding in larger tumours. The other diagnostic possibilities in this area include meningioma (*see* Case 60), and aneurysm (*see* Case 11).

Scan C shows a further lesion in another patient. Occasionally these tumours are bilateral.

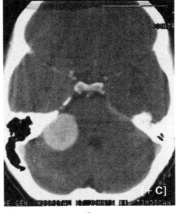

C

Case 59

Female, aged 63 years.

Seven-year history of numbness of right side of face and visual difficulty.

Right IIIrd and Vth cranial nerve palsies.

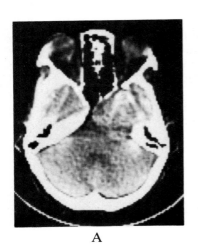

A

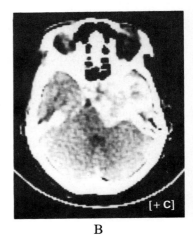

B

[+ C]

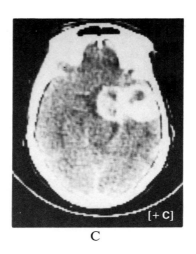

C

[+ C]

Case 59

Trigeminal neuroma

Scan A shows erosion of the apex of the right petrous bone. This is associated with a vague mass extending into the side of the sphenoid air sinus and the middle cranial fossa. Scans B and C show marked enhancement throughout this area and extending posteriorly to the cerebello-pontine angle, laterally into the temporal lobe and superiorly into the suprasellar cistern.

The long history suggests a benign lesion and the erosion of the petrous apex together with a lesion of the trigeminal nerve (Vth) suggests a trigeminal neuroma. This condition is very similar to an acoustic neuroma but lies more anteriorly at the skull base. The IIIrd nerve palsy is due to compression of this structure by the tumour lateral to the sphenoid sinus (in the cavernous sinus). Other possibilities include giant aneurysm (Case 14) or meningioma. Plain films and arteriography help to exclude these diagnoses. Metastatic disease frequently involves the skull base but the long history is against this.

Case 60

Female, aged 62 years.

Headaches. Cranial nerve palsies on the left.

Palsies of left IVth, Vth and VIth cranial nerves.

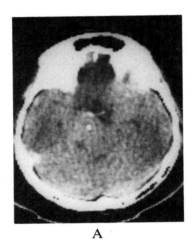

A

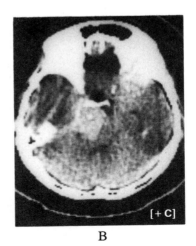

B

Case 60

Meningioma of posterior fossa

Scan A shows a vague area of increased density just to the left of the midline adjacent to the left cerebral peduncle. Two flecks of calcification are shown within it. Scan B at a slightly lower level shows marked enhancement in this well-defined lesion. It is seen to reach the dorsum sella anteriorly and to be displacing the fourth ventricle posteriorly. It also reaches postero-laterally almost as far as the cerebello-pontine angle.

This is a meningioma arising from the clivus and adjacent petrous bone. Meningiomas may be found anywhere around the margins of the posterior fossa including the cerebello-pontine angle, foramen magnum and the tentorium (*see* Cases 17 and 18). When they arise in the cerebello-pontine angle they invariably also reach the clivus and have a broader attachment to adjacent bone enabling them to be distinguished from acoustic tumours. Other possibilities here include a giant aneurysm of the basilar artery and trigeminal neuroma. Brain stem gliomas may rarely look like this. Plain films and arteriography may help to exclude these other diagnostic possibilities. Scan C shows a meningioma arising from the posterior tentorium (the bulk of it lies in the posterior fossa).

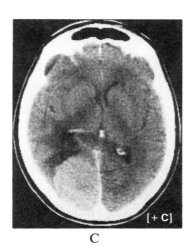

C

Case 61

Female, aged 8 years.

Occipital headache, vomiting, dizziness.

Bilateral papilloedema.

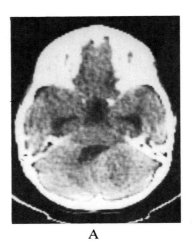

A

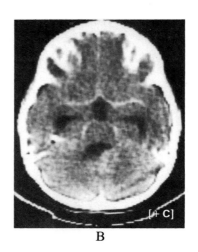

B

Case 61

Medulloblastoma

Scan A shows a dilated third ventricle and temporal horns. The fourth ventricle is compressed and deformed from the right side posteriorly. This is associated with a vague increased density in the area adjacent to the compression. Following contrast administration scan B shows there is some enhancement in this area.

The story and the appearances are consistent with a medulloblastoma. This tumour is confined to the posterior fossa and usually occurs in childhood. It arises in the vermis and invades the fourth ventricle and adjacent cerebellar hemispheres, as a result it is centrally placed. Such tumours are isodense with brain or of slightly raised density. They may show some calcification and areas of low density. They invariably enhance, though not dramatically.

The main differential diagnosis is ependymoma (*see* Case 62) and meningioma, although the latter is of necessity found around the margins of the posterior fossa. Choroid plexus papilloma is also a possibility, showing prominent enhancement (*see* Case 24).

A further example of medulloblastoma is shown below with calcification and low density (scans C and D).

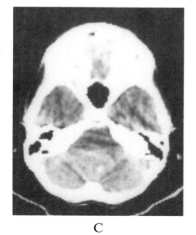

C

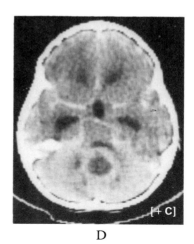

D

145

Case 62

Female, aged 78 years.

Vertigo and headaches for 6 months.

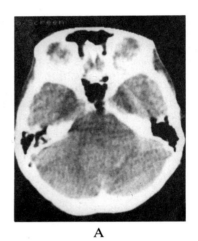

A

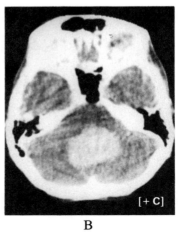

B

Case 62

Ependymoma

Scan A shows obliteration of the fourth ventricle and a vague area of increased density in the middle of the posterior fossa. Following contrast enhancement there is dramatic uptake of dye within the lesion (Scan B). Other slices showed hydrocephalus.

This lesion is an ependymoma. Such lesions arise from the linings of ventricles, usually the fourth, and produce obstruction to the ventricular outflow (hydrocephalus). They are found in a wider age group than medulloblastomas, but are common in young people. They are invariably slightly denser than surrounding brain. They may show calcification and usually have prominent enhancement (more so than medulloblastoma). They may be found in the third or lateral ventricles (*see* Case 21).

The differential diagnosis must include medulloblastoma (Case 61), meningioma (Case 60) and lymphoma (Case 19). The central position of an ependymoma is an important feature.

Case 63

Female, aged 37 years.

Vertigo, vomiting, headaches for 3 months.

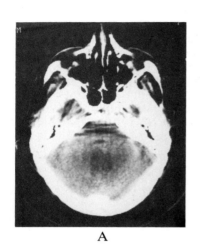

A

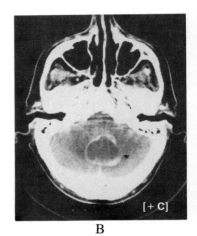

B

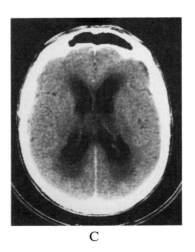

C

Case 63

Cystic astrocytoma (cerebellum)

Scan A shows a low density area in the vermis. This has compressed the fourth ventricle and displaced it forwards. Scan B shows a distinct ring of uptake after contrast enhancement. Scan C shows dilated ventricles with marked 'flare' around the ends of the ventricles (*see* Case 76).

This lesion is a cystic astrocytoma of the cerebellum. This condition is rather different from gliomas above the tentorium in that it is a much more benign process and invariably a cystic lesion. It is found in children and young adults and may be in the midline or laterally placed. Its low density and variable pattern of enhancement differentiate it from medulloblastoma (Case 61) and ependymoma (Case 62). The lesions with which it is most likely to be confused are haemangioblastoma (Case 64) and cerebellar infarction (Case 66).

Scan D shows a low density lesion expanding the brain stem anterior to the fourth ventricle. This is a glioma of the brain stem and is found in children. This process is similar to other gliomas and is more malignant than cerebellar astrocytoma.

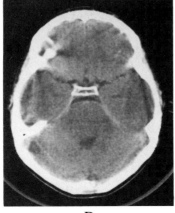

D

Case 64

Male, aged 30 years.

Headaches, nausea and vertigo for 2 months.

Papilloedema, nystagmus.

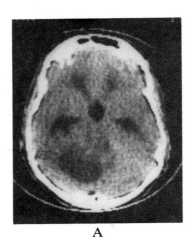

A

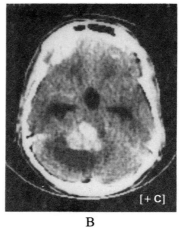

B

Case 64

Haemangioblastoma of cerebellum

Scan A shows a large cystic area in the upper left cerebellar hemisphere. The third and lateral ventricles are dilated. Following enhancement scan B shows a large densely enhancing nodule anteriorly in the cyst. The enhancing cystic nature of the lesion raises a few possibilities. This lesion is a haemangioblastoma—an uncommon benign tumour with a highly vascular nodule in the wall of the cyst. It is usually found in middle life. It tends to be found in the periphery of the cerebellum rather than centrally. The age group and the pattern of enhancement help to differentiate it from astrocytoma. A metastatic deposit is also a possibility. Angiography helps to show the characteristic highly vascular nodule which is usually smaller than this.

These tumours may be multiple and associated with retinal tumours (von Hippel–Lindau's syndrome).

Case 65

Female, aged 18 years.

Ten-year history of deafness, vertigo and swallowing problems.

Palsies of Vth, VIIth, VIIIth, IXth and Xth cranial nerves (left).

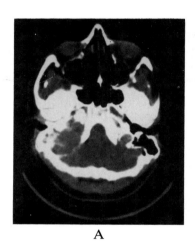

A

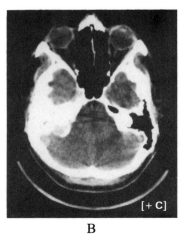

B

Case 65

Glomus jugulare tumour

Scan A has been taken close to the foramen magnum. There is dramatic bone destruction on the left side adjacent to the lower cerebellum. Compare this with normal bone detail on the right side. Scan B at a higher level shows enhancement extending into the left cerebellar hemisphere.

This lesion is compressing the pathways of many of the lower cranial nerves hence the multiple palsies. It is a tumour of the glomus jugulare. This arises within the jugular vein where it passes through the skull base. The degree of involvement of the cerebello-pontine angle and cerebellum is variable. Although benign, it is highly vascular and difficult to remove.

The main differentials here must be metastatic deposits in the skull base, meningioma, and rarely chordoma (usually anteriorly placed on the clivus). A neuroma of the lower cranial nerves is also a possibility.

Case 66

Female, aged 59 years.

Sudden onset of headache and vomiting.

Severe nystagmus.

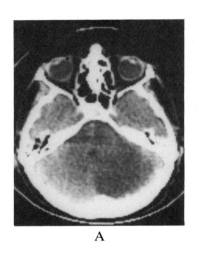

A

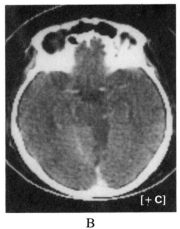

B

Case 66

Cerebellar infarction

Scan A shows a low density area in the right cerebellar hemisphere with some displacement of the fourth ventricle to the left. After contrast enhancement scan B was taken at a higher level and shows the apex of the cerebellum surrounded by the upper tentorium which is 'U'-shaped. The right side of the upper cerebellum is also of low density. The lesion does not enhance.

The pattern is non-specific but the clearcut involvement of the upper cerebellar hemisphere in this way is very suggestive of an infarct in the territory of the superior cerebellar artery. This is much less common than infarction in the cerebral hemispheres. Because it occurs in the confined space of the posterior fossa a mass effect is more common. Enhancement is usually absent. Only the history of sudden onset differentiates it from a cystic astrocytoma.

Case 67

Female, aged 25 years.

Three-year history of amenorrhoea. Galactorrhoea.

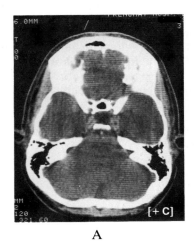

A

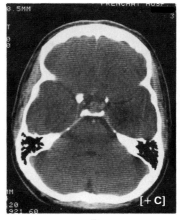

B

Case 67

Pituitary adenoma

Scan A shows a low density area in the pituitary fossa which is mildly enlarged, particularly on the right side. This scan was taken with contrast medium enhancement and the raised density areas on either side of the fossa are due to the normal cavernous sinus. At a slightly higher level scan B shows a small area of enhancement in the pituitary fossa. This appearance is due to an adenoma of the pituitary gland. These benign tumours are common and may produce increased hormone production, e.g. acromegaly or hyperprolactin states (as in this case). Many do not secrete hormones however but present with hypopituitarism, headache or visual problems (as the tumour grows up out of the fossa and presses on the optic chiasm). Adenomas present a variety of appearances and may contain densities between calcification and cyst fluid (as in this case). Enhancement is variable but should always be looked for.

The tumours may be of considerable size by the time they present. They may extend laterally and upwards. Scan C shows a case with visual failure and some lateral extension. Scan D shows a big cystic tumour extending to the top of the third ventricle and producing hydrocephalus. (For the differential diagnosis *see* Cases 68, 69 and 70).

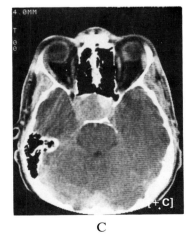

C

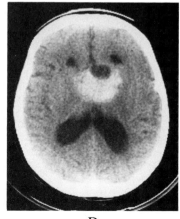

D

Case 68

Female, aged 19 years.

Headache and visual failure for 2 years.

Bitemporal hemianopia.

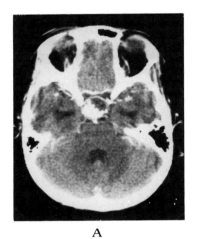

A

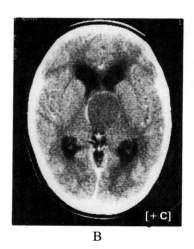

B

Case 68

Craniopharyngioma

Scan A shows irregular calcification in the posterior part of the pituitary fossa on the left. The fossa is enlarged. Scan B with enhancement shows the lesion extending up into the expected position of the third ventricle which has been obliterated. The lesion is well defined and of low density, suggesting fluid. Having reached the level of the foramen of Munro, it has caused dilatation of the lateral ventricles. There is enhancement of the left lateral edge of the lesion.

The combination of calcification, cystic component and marginal enhancement in a suprasellar lesion is diagnostic of craniopharyngioma. This tumour is developmental in origin and arises in the pituitary fossa or suprasellar area. It is benign and usually contains brown oily fluid. Such tumours are usually seen in children and young adults, but may occasionally go unnoticed until later life.

The main differentials are pituitary adenoma (calcification much less common, Case 67) and optic chiasm glioma (calcification and cystic change unusual, Case 69).

Case 69

Female, aged 13 years.

Headaches and increasing blindness for 3 months.

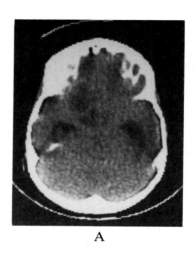

A

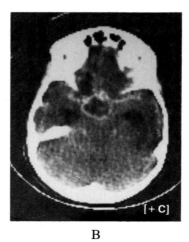

B

Case 69

Glioma of the optic chiasm

Scan A shows dilated temporal horns of the lateral ventricles and a vague low density area in the midline just above the pituitary fossa. On another slice the pituitary fossa was mildly enlarged. Scan B shows an irregular ring-like area of enhancement in the suprasellar area (the lines running laterally from this are the normal middle cerebral arteries).

The diagnostic possibilities include pituitary tumours, craniopharyngioma, tumours of the floor of the third ventricle (hypothalamus) or optic chiasm. Plain X-rays of the skull showed widening of optic foramina consistent with an abnormality of the optic nerves. This lesion is a glioma of the optic chiasm. It is a tumour of variable malignancy and found mostly in children. Some lesions are confined to the orbit and others are associated with multiple neurofibromas.

Male, aged 62 years.

Gradual visual loss for 2 years.

Bitemporal hemianopia.

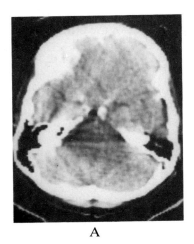

A

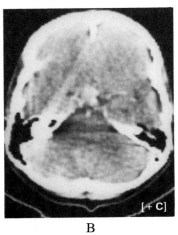

B

Case 70

Suprasellar aneurysm

Scan A shows a vague suggestion of a mass in the upper pituitary fossa and suprasellar cistern. After enhancement scan B shows this lesion to be taking up dye.

The appearances are non-specific and would certainly do for a pituitary adenoma but the pituitary fossa was normal on plain films. There is no calcification or cystic change to suggest a craniopharyngioma. A tumour of the optic chiasm such as a glioma or neurofibroma would certainly have to be considered.

Angiography showed this to be an aneurysm arising from the carotid siphon. This is an important possibility in any suprasellar lesion and angiography is advisable in many cases of suspected pituitary and suprasellar tumours.

Case 71

Male, aged 39 years.

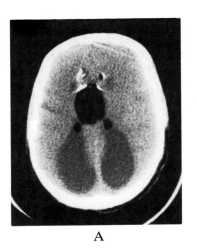

A

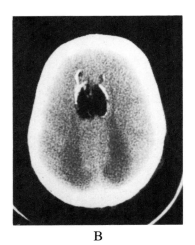

B

Case 71

Lipoma of corpus callosum

Scan A shows dilated lateral ventricles separated anteriorly by a well circumscribed lesion of very low density with some marginal calcification. Scan B shows a higher level where the calcification is seen to follow the lateral margin of the lesion which clearly lies in the corpus callosum. There was no change after contrast enhancement. Density measurements confirmed the presence of fat, but usually this density could easily be due to air (*see* Case 72).

The lesion is typical of a lipoma of the corpus callosum. This is a benign tumour of developmental origin with a high fat content which may go unnoticed or be associated with partial absence (agenesis) of the corpus callosum. The calcified rim is typical and is often seen on plain skull films.

Other very low density fatty tumours occur in the brain such as dermoids and epidermoids (cholesteatoma or pearly tumour). These do not usually calcify and tend to lie in the midline along the floor of the third ventricle (*see* scan C) or in the cerebello-pontine angle. Fat is also seen in some hamartomas (*see* Case 57).

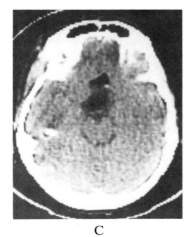

C

Case 72

Female, aged 71 years.

Clear fluid running from nose following pituitary surgery.

CSF rhinorrhoea.

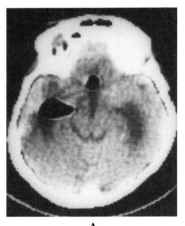

A

Case 72

Intracranial air (pneumocephalus)

Scan A shows areas of very low density in a dilated left temporal horn and in the anterior third ventricle. Density measurement showed this to be air not fat, and it is clearly within the ventricular system. The patient had recently undergone pituitary surgery via the nose and an uncommon complication of this is associated perforation of the floor of the third ventricle. The floor of the pituitary fossa did not heal and allowed air from the nasal cavity to enter the subarachnoid and ventricular spaces.

This appearance may also be seen following any craniotomy, and in head trauma where fractures of the skull base have allowed air from the paranasal sinuses to enter the cranial cavity. In this latter situation CSF leaks and even meningitis may follow.

Case 73

Female, aged 17 years.

Large head since infancy.

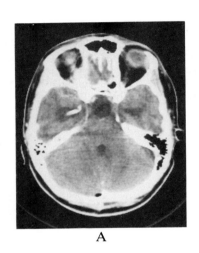

A

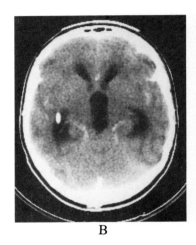

B

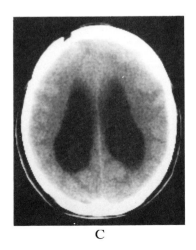

C

Case 73

Aqueduct stenosis

Scan A shows a normal-sized fourth ventricle. The region over the pituitary fossa is of unusually low density. This is due to downward bulging of the dilated third ventricle visible on scan B. Also of note is a density in the dilated left temporal horn. This is due to a shunt. Scans B and C show dilated third and lateral ventricles. There was no change after contrast enhancement.

The combination of a normal fourth ventricle with dilated third and lateral ventricles is consistent with a block of the aqueduct. This may be due to a tumour in this area such as a pinealoma (*see* Case 23) or meningioma of the tentorium. In this case there is no evidence for this and the hydrocephalus is due to a congenital narrowing of the aqueduct.

Case 74

Male, aged 3 months.

Increasing head circumference since birth.

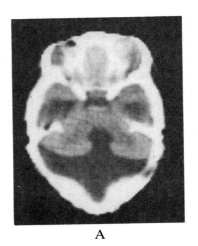

A

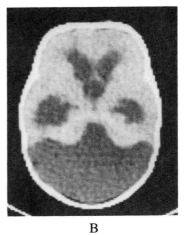

B

Case 74

Dandy–Walker syndrome

Scan A shows a dilated fourth ventricle communicating posteriorly through an abnormally wide channel to a hugely dilated cisterna magna. Scan B shows this latter structure extending up into the area below the tentorium, which is pushed upwards. The third and lateral ventricles are markedly dilated. In any case of hydrocephalus it is essential to examine all the ventricles to identify the level of the block, e.g. lateral ventricles only dilated if block at foramen of Munro (*see* Case 68), third and lateral ventricles dilated in blocks at the back of the third ventricle pinealoma (Case 23) or aqueduct stenosis (Case 73), etc. In this case, since the fourth is dilated, clearly the block must be distal to this structure in the basal cisterns or beyond. Dandy-Walker syndrome is caused by congenital blockage of the exit foramina of the fourth ventricle and improper development of the vermis which allows CSF to accumulate in this vast cisterna magna. The fourth ventricle and cistern may be continuous in some cases.

See also Cases 73, 75 and 76.

Case 75

Male, aged 2 years.

Increasing head circumference since birth.

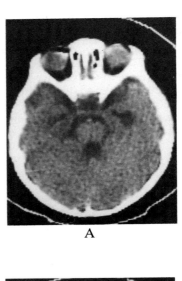

A

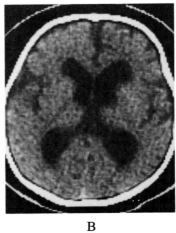

B

Case 75

Communicating hydrocephalus

Scan A shows dilatation of the fourth ventricle, the temporal horns and the basal cisterns. Scan B shows dilatation of the third and lateral ventricles and CSF spaces over the cortex.

If this was an adult patient the appearances might be confused with cerebral atrophy (*see* Case 78). This condition is rare in children and then is associated with extensive white matter disease (*see* Case 38). In addition, the presence of dilated temporal horns and a sharp angle between the frontal horns of the lateral ventricles are features that argue against atrophy.

This appearance is due to communicating hydrocephalus. This is a common cause of an enlarged head in childhood and is due to obstruction to the passage of CSF in the basal cisterns or over the hemispheres as it passes to be resorbed along the sagittal sinus. Consequently all the ventricles will be dilated and also to some extent the basal cisterns and the spaces over the cortex depending on the level of obstruction. This process is caused by birth injury with blood in the CSF, or as a result of meningitis (*see* Cases 73, 74, 76).

Case 76

Male, aged 75 years.

Slowly increasing dementia, ataxia and incontinence.

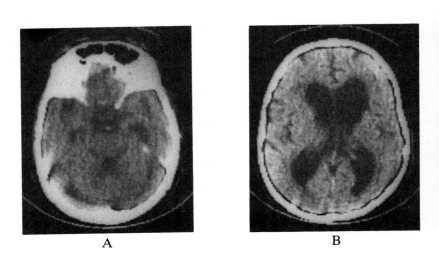

A   B

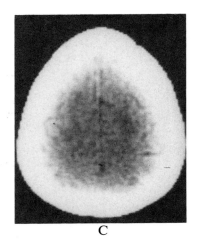

C

Case 76

Normal pressure hydrocephalus

Scan A shows dilatation of the fourth ventricle and temporal horns. Scan B shows dilated third and lateral ventricles. There is a little excess fluid in the basal cisterns and over the lower hemispheres. Scan C shows no significant atrophy at the vertex.

As in Case 75, the appearances are similar to those of atrophy except the dilatation of the ventricles is out of proportion to the degree of sulcal widening (*see* Case 78). Also the angle between the frontal horns is acute which favours hydrocephalus rather than an obtuse angle as seen in atrophy.

In older patients this kind of hydrocephalus is often insidious and clinically appears like cerebral atrophy, but the added features of incontinence and ataxia suggest hydrocephalus. At this stage there is usually no raised pressure within the ventricle hence the term 'normal pressure'. It is important to suspect this diagnosis as some patients' dementia can be reversed by shunting. The diagnosis can be confirmed using flow studies of contrast medium in the CSF.

Hydrocephalus is also seen in many acute states as the result of meningitis or subarachnoid haemorrhage. Certain tumours block the CSF pathways and produce hydrocephalus. These acute types of hydrocephalus may show a low density flare around the ends of the lateral ventricles (*see* Case 63).

Female, aged 49 years.

Three-week history of headache and fever.

Deeply comatose.

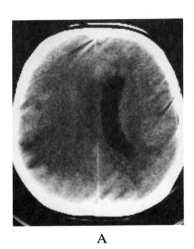

A

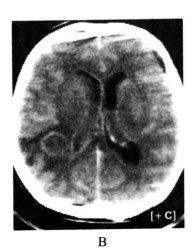

B

Case 77

Ventriculitis

Scan A shows an ill-defined low density area in the left parietal region due to cerebral oedema. The adjacent ventricle is more opaque than on the other side. Both ventricles are mildly dilated. Scan B shows a ring-like area of enhancement in the area of oedema. The left ventricle is outlined by a fine rim of enhancement. This is most evident in the frontal horn (compare with normal right side). Both scans show diagonal streaks due to patient movement.

The lesion in the left parietal region is an abscess. The appearance in the left ventricle is due to inflammation along the lining of the ventricle (ependyma) and the CSF within it is denser than usual due to pus. These features should be looked for in any ill patient as ventriculitis has a high mortality. At post mortem the abscess was found to have ruptured into the left ventricle.

Case 78

Male, aged 68 years.

Progressive dementia over 3 years.

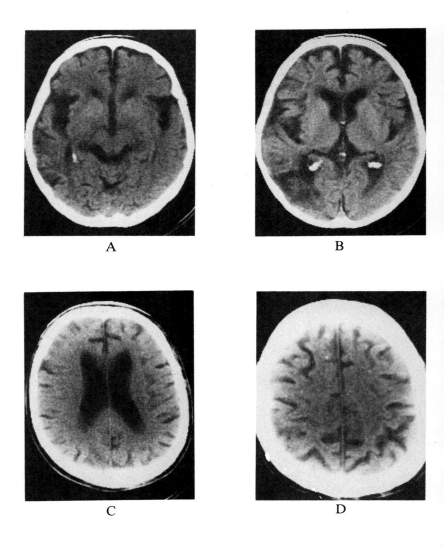

A

B

C

D

Case 78

Cerebral atrophy

Scan A shows dramatic widening of the sylvian fissures (not to be confused with temporal horns which are lower in position and a different shape, *see* Case 73). The subarachnoid spaces over the hemispheres and behind the brain stem (quadrigeminal cistern) are also dilated. The third ventricle is not particularly dilated. Scan B shows mildly dilated lateral ventricles with a flat angle between the frontal horns. The inter-hemispheral fissure is also wide. Scan C shows the dilated lateral ventricles and widened sulci and scan D shows widened sulci over the vertex.

The appearances are those of cerebral atrophy. This may be a normal finding with increasing age but is excessive for a patient of this age. In this patient it represents the commonest form of presenile dementia, called 'Alzheimer's disease'. The degree of sulcal widening is not always proportional to the extent of the intellectual loss, but ventricular dilatation does correlate quite well. The ratio of ventricular size to sulcal widening is appropriate unlike hydrocephalus. For other differential diagnoses *see* Cases 73, 74, 75 and 76. Multiple infarcts are described in Case 39. (These can mimic Alzheimer's disease clinically and are often found in association with atrophy.)

Case 79

Female, aged 67 years.

Gradually increasing ataxia for 4 years.

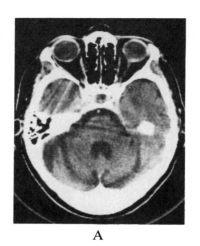

A

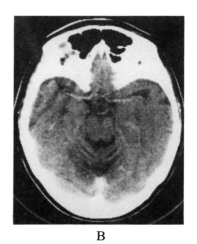

B

Case 79

Cerebellar atrophy

Scan A shows widening of the subarachnoid spaces in the posterior fossa including the cerebello-pontine angle. Scan B shows dramatic widening of the spaces over the upper cerebellum to an extent that the cerebellar folia are clearly outlined. The changes are limited by the tentorium on either side.

These changes are similar to those in Case 78 except that they are present in the cerebellum. The supratentorial area is not involved. This is due to cerebellar atrophy—an uncommon condition usually distinct from cerebral atrophy. There are a number of different causes. Alcoholism may be involved.

Case 80

Female, aged 43 years.

Right-sided focal epilepsy.

Right hemiparesis.

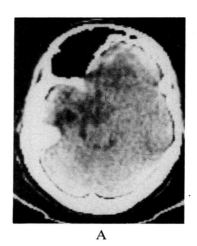

A

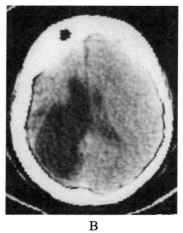

B

Case 80

Hemi-atrophy

Scan A shows dilatation of the left frontal sinus, elevation of the left petrous bone and some enlargement of the left temporal horn. Scan B shows some shift of midline structures to the left with dilatation of the left ventricle particularly posteriorly. There is also marked thickening of the vault on the left.

The changes imply loss of volume in the left cerebral hemisphere (hemi-atrophy). The patient had severe encephalitis as a child. There was obviously extensive damage to the left hemisphere at that time and it did not subsequently develop normally. As a result, the bony structures on this side have enlarged to accommodate the loss of brain substance. Such a response is usually only seen following brain damage occurring in childhood when the tissues are still growing.

Case 81

Male, aged 64 years.

Headache, right-sided weakness for 10 days.

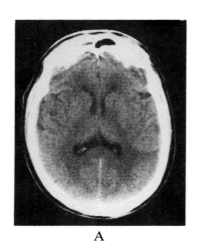

A

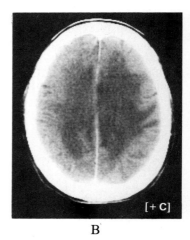

[+ C]

B

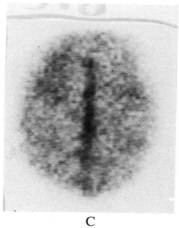

C

Case 81

Cerebral oedema (sagittal sinus thrombosis)

Scan A shows small ventricles for a patient of this age, suggesting a generalized increase in intracranial pressure. There is no shift. After enhancement scan B shows low density areas due to swelling in the upper part of both hemispheres. There were no abnormal areas of enhancement.

The findings are those of cerebral oedema. This may be due to a variety of toxic conditions, trauma, etc. Bilateral isodense chronic subdurals may give a similar appearance. In this instance further tests revealed thrombosis of the superior sagittal sinus. Scan C, a dynamic isotope scan over the vertex, shows irregular filling of the sagittal sinus consistent with this diagnosis. A generalized cerebral oedema results. The condition is related to venous infarction (*see* Case 33). The CT scan cannot be relied on to show the sagittal sinus accurately as the falx obscures the sinus.

Scan D shows generalized cerebral swelling in a 65-year-old following trauma. The ventricles are compressed and there is a vague low density area in the white matter of both hemispheres.

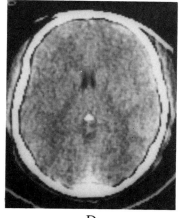

D

Case 82

Female, aged 45 years.

Headache for 10 months.

Papilloedema.

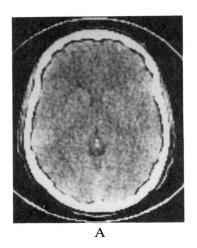

A

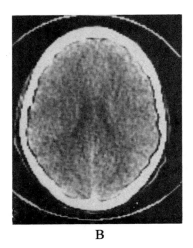

B

Case 82

Benign intracranial hypertension

Scan A shows unusually small ventricles for a patient of this age. Scan B confirms this at a higher level showing the bodies of the lateral ventricles. There was no change after contrast enhancement.

The changes suggest generalized cerebral swelling although there are no changes in the white matter (*see* Case 81). The differential diagnosis must include bilateral isodense subdurals, sinus thrombosis, etc., but there was no evidence of these on other tests.

This condition, also known as 'pseudo-tumour cerebri' is characterized by headache and papilloedema. It is of unknown origin but may be associated with certain systemic diseases. It is usually seen in women.

Male, aged 73 years.

Increasing unsteadiness and weakness.

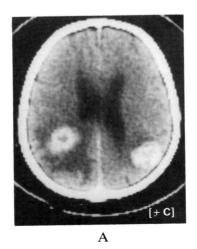

A

Case 83

Multiple metastases

Scan A shows one large enhancing lesion in each hemisphere. These are surrounded by a zone of oedema.

Multiple lesions raise a fairly limited range of diagnostic possibilities. Metastases and infarcts are the most common and these follow the pattern of their pathologies as described elsewhere (*see* Cases 20 and 39). Multiple abscesses are usually ring-like (*see* Case 85). Neurofibromas are usually found along the course of cranial nerves and so are seen at the skull base (*see* Case 84). Multiple meningiomas have the usual characteristics of meningiomas as described elsewhere. They are usually confined to the margins of the brain wherever dura is found (*see* Cases 17 and 86).

Case 84

Male, aged 32 years.

Decreasing vision and proptosis in right eye.

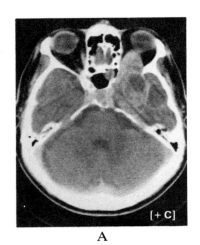

A

Case 84

Multiple neurofibromas

Scan A shows a multilobular enhancing mass in the right middle fossa extending forwards into the back of the right orbit. In some areas the lesion looks cystic.

A lesion running into the back of the orbit like this is likely to be a neuroma of the optic or related nerve; or a glioma of the optic nerve or optic chiasm. The history dated back 6 years indicating a basically benign process such as a neuroma rather than a glioma.

Neurofibromas occur along the line of cranial nerves and so are found in this area where the IInd, IIIrd, IVth, and VIth cranial nerves run; at the apex of the petrous bone in the Vth nerve (*see* Case 59); and in the cerebello-pontine angle as VIIIth (acoustic) nerve tumours (*see* Case 58). The degree of enhancement is usually moderate.

Case 85

Female, aged 30 years.

Increasing headache and confusion.

Multiple neurological deficits, fever, papilloedema.

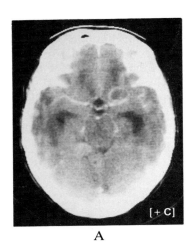

A

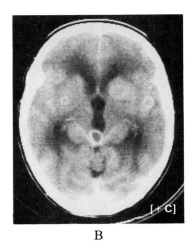

B

Case 85

Multiple abscesses

Scan A shows dilated temporal horns. An enhancing ring shadow is shown in the right temporal region just anterior to the right middle cerebral artery. Also with contrast enhancement scan B shows several ring shadows in both hemispheres. The ventricles are dilated.

These lesions are typical of abscesses but metastases are often also ring-shaped. The presence of fever and leucocytosis help to distinguish them. Multiple granulomas such as tuberculomas are also a possibility (*see* Case 25). Multiple abscesses are usually due to septicaemia.

Some abscesses become confluent and may mimic a glioma (*see* front cover).

Case 86

Male, aged 62 years.

Headaches for 2 years.

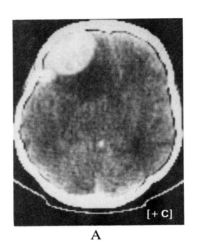

A

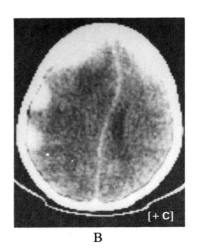

B

Case 86

Multiple meningiomas

Scan A shows a well-defined densely enhancing mass adjacent to the left frontal bone. There is a suggestion of a smaller further lesion just behind it. Scan B shows two further similar lesions also under the vault at a higher level and more posteriorly placed. There is marked compression and displacement of the ventricles.

These lesions have all the features of meningiomas (*see* Case 17). Meningiomas are not uncommonly multiple and are invariably peripherally sited. The major differentials are metastases (*see* Case 83), neurofibromas (*see* Case 84) and granulomas (*see* Case 25).

Suggested further reading

1. Ambrose J. (1973) 'Computerized transverse axial scanning (tomography). Part 2. Clinical applications.' *British Journal of Radiology*, **46**, 1023-47.
2. Burrows E.H. and Leeds N.E. (1981) *Neuroradiology*. Churchill Livingstone, New York.
3. Harwood-Nash D. and Fitz C.R. (1976) *Neuroradiology in Infants and Children*. Mosby Co., St Louis, Vol. 2.
4. Hounsfield G.N. (1973) 'Computerized transverse axial scanning (tomography). Part 1. Description of system.' *British Journal of Radiology*, **46**, 1016-22.
5. Sutton D. (ed) (1980) 'CT scanning CNS 1-2.' *A Textbook of Radiology and Imaging* (3rd ed). Vol 2, Chapters 63 and 64. Churchill Livingstone, Edinburgh.

Pathology index